RADIONICS
AND THE
SUBTLE ANATOMY OF MAN

RADIONICS AND THE SUBTLE ANATOMY OF MAN

by

DAVID V. TANSLEY, D.C.

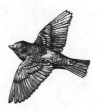

THE C. W. DANIEL COMPANY LIMITED
1 Church Path, Saffron Walden, Essex, United Kingdom

First published August 1972
Second Impression February 1974
Third Impression February 1976
Fourth Impression October 1980
Fifth Impression September 1982
Sixth Impression May 1985
Seventh Impression June 1988
Eighth Impression May 1993
Ninth Impression October 1998

ISBN 0 85032 089 5

Printed in Great Britain by
Hillman Printers (Frome) Ltd, Frome, Somerset

INTRODUCTION

If one examines the history and development of radionics from the pioneering work of Dr. Albert Abrams and Ruth Drown, to the latest experimental work at the de la Warr Laboratories, a curious paradox emerges.

Radionics professes to be a method of diagnosis and therapy, which is primarily concerned with the utilization of subtle force fields and energies, for the purpose of investigating and combating the causes of disease which ravage humanity and the other kingdoms of nature. However, in discussions or articles, in the methods of diagnosis and treatment, and in the rate books which provide the very core of radionic therapeutic measures, one finds continual reference to the physical organic systems of man, and precious little of practical value regarding the probability of underlying force fields which might govern and determine the health of the physical form.

It would seem that this unfortunate paradox has emerged because radionics, which is essentially a paraphysical method of diagnosis and treatment, utilizing the faculty of extra-sensory perception and the concept of 'action at a distance', has predicated its approach to the problems of disease upon a semi-orthodox terminology and rationale.

There can be no doubt that it was necessary for Abrams to lay the foundation for radionics in terms of physical reference, after all, he was a physician and his training and discipline required this of him. Surely it was revolutionary enough that he discarded the cell theory of disease, and replaced it with the electron theory. Disease to him was not a matter so crude as cell dysfunction, but had a subtler nuance in that it was related to what he felt was the ultimate divisibility of matter. By moving away from a purely physical approach to disease, Abrams showed that the cause of disease can be traced sequentially to more and more subtle realms. This trend is also expressed in the fields of diagnosis and, eventually, treatment.

Although both Abrams and Drown treated their patients by means of direct attachment to the instrument, in much the same way as a physiotherapist would apply galvanic or diathermy modalities, there are references in their writings, even in those early days, which show that diagnosis and treatment at a distance were not only considered, but carried out with effective results. I am going to relate them here, because the sequence, if carried to its logical conclusion, leads us ultimately to consider the possibility of utilizing radionic diagnostic and therapeutic techniques in the light of knowledge derived from the ancient teachings of the East.

Abrams relates that he evolved from working directly with the patient or patient's blood spot, to a diagnostic technique which involved using the earth itself as a conducting medium for pathological energy. This method which he called radiogeodiagnosis proved suitable over short distances but only partially successful over long distances.

He then experimented with telediagnosis which utilized the overhead telephone wires to link him with the patient sample. This sample would be placed near the phone in another physician's office, and Abrams would diagnose the case at a distance. His results and their accuracy were confirmed by laboratory tests. Experiments were effectively carried out for distances in excess of five hundred miles. Abrams concluded that pathological energy could be conveyed over long distances by means of telephone wires.

This eventually led to what Abrams referred to as teleaerodiagnosis, in which there was no visible connection with the patient at all. He succeeded in recognizing energy patterns of disease by aerial transmission over a distance of one mile, with the observation that much more experimentation along such lines would be needed, to enable him to exceed that distance.

Through the process of repeated experiments Abrams

refined his techniques of diagnosis, progressing from direct physical contact between the patient and the instrument, to the utilization of the ethers as a connecting medium.

The chiropractor Ruth Drown was to carry this concept into the application of treatment at a distance, and the term 'broadcasting' found a niche in radionic parlance. In 1933 this technique was in its infancy, but as Drown points out, many vital cases were healed through this method.

Since 1933 radionics has developed and refined the techniques of diagnosis and treatment at a distance. Today every practitioner uses these methods as a standard procedure. What Abrams and Drown may have seen as unusual, the modern radionic therapist accepts as commonplace. The credit for this must surely go to the untiring efforts of the late George de la Warr and his wife, at their laboratories in Oxford.

Despite the necessary refinement of techniques and instrumentation over the past twenty-five years, there is a nagging suspicion in my mind that the key implication in the discovery by Abrams and Drown, of diagnosis and treatment at a distance, has been missed.

I believe that they pointed the way as far back as 1924, to the concept that man has a body of highly attenuated matter, which he derives from the energy field in the earth, and which links him with all life. This body is referred to in Eastern literature as the etheric body.

Today, most if not all radionic practitioners would agree that it is their belief that man does have what is referred to as an etheric body. The remarkable thing is that the matter is allowed to rest right there, and the practitioner continues to diagnose and treat in terms of cellular pathology and organic systems.

Inherent in the fact that Abrams diagnosed at a distance, and Drown treated absent patients, is an implication that I find of great interest. It is this. Each of them in their own way broke away from the use of the electromagnetic field and began to utilize an energy field of a more subtle nature. Their actions suggest that they were using the etheric force field of the earth as a connecting medium between them and their patients. By doing this they indicated that man need no longer be looked upon as a fortuitous conglomeration of organ systems, but something more subtle.

Man is a series of high frequency energy systems which integrate him into the universal scheme of things. These systems have an anatomy and physiology of their own, which in the final analysis determine the appearance and activity of the physical form, and diagnosis and treatment can be based upon this fact. Abrams and Drown launched this concept, but we have been content to swim along the shoreline ever since, not daring for various reasons to strike out into uncharted waters.

I feel very strongly that the time has come for radionics to bear witness to the subtle anatomy of man; this I believe to be its innate purpose. Radionics by its very nature is related to the laws and principles that govern the etheric, emotional and mental levels of existence, therefore new techniques of diagnosis and treatment based on these laws and principles should render the practitioner more effective in his work.

The sequence of Abrams' approach to healing can be stated so.

Physical   Atomic
Cell Theory   Electron Theory

I suggest that this sequence can be extended in the following manner.

Physical   Atomic
Cell Theory   Electron Theory   Etheric

In departing, then, from a physically orientated approach to radionics, it is necessary to accept as a working hypothesis the existence of three basic factors.

First   The actuality of the etheric formative forces which permeate all space and every form living therein, be it a human being or a planet.

Second   That man has a subtle anatomy which relates him to the forces in his immediate environment, and to those of the universe at large, and upon which the physical form is totally dependent for its expression of Life.

Third   That any imbalance in the reciprocal interplay of energies between the various aspects of man's subtle anatomy, or between man and the surrounding forces, results in dis-ease.

These three basic factors provide the framework for a new radionic approach to health, one that is fast, simple and above all effective. It eliminates the welter of inconsequential details that can arise during the course of a physically orientated radionic diagnosis, because it considers man from a holistic, not a fragmentary point of view.

The purpose of this book is to provide a simple yet practical outline of the subtle anatomy of man, and to explore techniques of diagnosis and treatment based on this information. Dr. H. Tomlinson, in his book *The Divination of Disease*, wrote: 'The treatment of one of the metaphysical bodies alone, opens up a very fascinating future work.'

What follows will, I hope, prove the substance of his words, and encourage other radionic practitioners to explore the same pathways, leading to a deeper understanding of their inner beings, for from this knowledge comes effectiveness in the field of healing.

ACKNOWLEDGMENTS

I wish to express my sincere thanks to the following for permission to quote from various works:

The Rudolf Steiner Press: *The Etheric Formative Forces in Cosmos, Earth and Man* by Guenther Wachsmuth. *Physical and Ethereal Spaces* by George Adams. The Lucis Press: *Treatise on Cosmic Fire and Esoteric Healing* by Alice A. Bailey. C.W. Daniel Co. Ltd. *The Twelve Healers and Other Remedies* by Dr. Edward Bach. I also acknowledge my indebtedness for the quotations used from *Space and The Light of The Creation*, written and privately published by George Adams. Jonathan Cape: *Ideas and Integrities* by R. Buckminster Fuller. My special thanks to Dr. A.K. Bhattacharya of Naihati, West Bengal for his interest in my work and for permission to quote from *Gem Therapy* written by his late father Dr. B. Bhattacharya (Firma K.L. Mukhopadhyay, Calcutta). Finally I would like to express my gratitude to John Wilcox, author of *Radionics in Theory and Practice*, for his help with this manuscript in its formative stages.

THIS BOOK IS DEDICATED TO THE MEMORY OF

Dr. Albert Abrams
Dr. Ruth Drown, D.C.
and
George de la Warr
Pioneers in the field of radionics.

And to those who serve in the various
healing arts with an open heart and mind.

CONTENTS

		Page
1.	The Esoteric Constitution of Man	13
2.	The Etheric Body	17
3.	The Force Centres	23
4.	The Seven Major Spinal Chakras	32
5.	Vitality and the Dynamics of Pranic Reception	49
6.	The Centre Therapy Instrument	58
7.	Diagnosis and the Subtle Bodies	66
8.	Centre Therapy	76
9.	Etherialized Medicines	87
10.	The Future Trend	93

CHAPTER ONE

THE ESOTERIC CONSTITUTION OF MAN

The mere looking at externals is a matter for clowns, but the intuition of internals is a secret which belongs to physicians.

Paracelsus

Since ancient times man has held the belief that his physical body is simply the externalization of more subtle vehicles of manifestation. References to these invisible bodies are to be found in a wide variety of texts originating in China, India, Egypt and ancient Greece. The Bible too refers frequently to the subtle anatomy of man, particularly in *The Revelation of St. John*.

It is fashionable today to dismiss such ancient beliefs as mere superstition, holding them as impracticable and beyond any scientific proof. Curiously enough many of these writings, some of which are over five thousand years old, show clearly that the ancient seers and philosophers had a remarkably detailed knowledge of the anatomy and physiology of the human nervous and endocrine systems — two areas in which modern science still has much to learn.

For the most part, radionic practitioners accept that man has a subtle anatomy, but there are few who view it as they would the physical body, that is, as having definite form and clearly defined functions. It tends to become a rather vague amorphous mass into which healing rates are projected, and practitioners place a limit on their effectiveness by using this approach.

There is a passage in Wachsmuth's book *The Etheric Formative Forces in Cosmos, Earth and Man*, which is relevant to this point. He writes:

> In future the art of healing will rest upon a knowledge of the etheric in Nature and in man . . . If one views these realities not abstractly, but in the living man in their world relationship, one then arrives at new forms of knowledge in pathology and therapy in the art of healing.

This passage not only indicates the future trend of the healing arts when they emerge from the present materialism, but clearly shows that the reality of the etheric forces and the subtle workings of nature must not be viewed in a pseudo-mystical manner, but in a practical context relevant to the living man. The vague idea of the subtle bodies underlying the physical form must be replaced with the knowledge of structures which have a definite relationship to the visible anatomy and its physiological processes.

What now follows is an outline of the sevenfold nature of man, and the planes of matter upon which various aspects of his being are found. It is not intended as the final word, but put forward as a working hypothesis. Should the reader care to follow this line of thought more deeply, there is ample material to study in the esoteric literature available today. The purpose of this outline is to provide a picture of the subtle bodies of man in their universal context, and replace the 'amorphous mass' approach with something inherently more practical and close to reality.

The seven planes upon which man is said to have his being are listed as follows, from above downwards. The first or Divine plane; the second or Monadic plane; the third or Spiritual plane; the fourth or Intuitional plane; the fifth or Mental plane; the sixth or Emotional plane; the seventh or Physical plane.

Each of these planes is subdivided into what are known as seven sub-planes, giving a total of forty-nine planes in all. The highest aspect of man is found upon the monadic plane. This aspect uses the soul as its vehicle of expression, which is found upon the higher mental planes. The soul in its turn utilizes the lower self in order to gain experience in the three worlds of the lower mental planes, the emotional plane and the physical plane.

In other words man manifests as a triplicity of spirit, soul and body. The pure spirit is analogous to the Father in heaven, the soul is the high self, and the body the low self. The low self is likewise triple in nature, consisting of the mental body, the emotional or astral body, and the physical-etheric body.

The low self may in fact be considered as a quaternary if the

The Seven Planes and Man's Subtle Anatomy

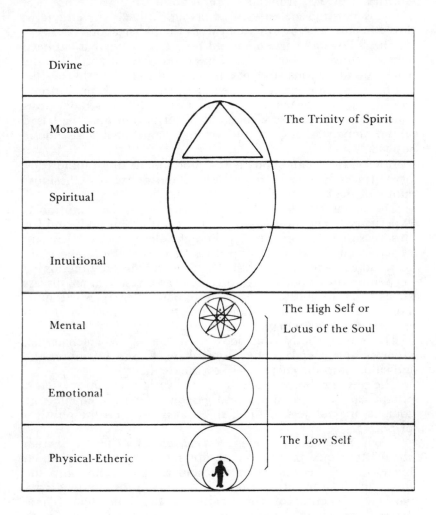

Divine

Monadic   The Trinity of Spirit

Spiritual

Intuitional

Mental   The High Self or
                                           Lotus of the Soul

Emotional

Physical-Etheric   The Low Self

physical and etheric bodies are looked upon as separate entities. However from an esoteric point of view the physical body is not considered as a principle, whereas the etheric is. For our purposes the etheric body is the physical body.

The following diagram should help to clarify what has been written above. This brief detail has been given just to fill in the background; serious students are advised to follow this outline up from the appropriate writings. For the radionic practitioner who is only interested in it for practical utilization in diagnosis and treatment, then the focus of his attention must be based in an understanding of the mental, emotional and etheric aspects.

Briefly, the mental body is that body made up of mind stuff or chitta as it is called in Eastern philosophy. It is the most subtle of the bodies utilized by the soul.

The astral vehicle is that body through which emotion is experienced. The interplay of desire is felt in this body and for this reason it is sometimes called the desire body. Here are experienced the pairs of opposites such as pleasure and pain, fear and courage and so forth. Most individuals are functioning very potently through this body, and as a result much disease stems from the constant chaotic interplay of energies within it. For this reason the radionic practitioner must come to understand its workings.

The etheric body, the densest of the subtle mechanisms, vitalizes and energizes the physical body, and integrates the individual into the energy field of the earth.

The physical body, made up of the various organic systems, comprised of dense, liquid and gaseous materials, enables the soul, in the fullness of time, to express itself on the physical plane.

When St. John wrote in *Revelation* of 'The city which stands foursquare', he was describing those energies which make up the mechanism of the soul as it descends into the force field of the earth, and each expression of energy carries with it a picture of the health of the individual. These emanations tell the radionic practitioner what is wrong with his patient, therefore the more knowledge the practitioner has of the subtle anatomy of man, the more effective he is going to be in his art.

CHAPTER TWO

THE ETHERIC BODY

In the study of the etheric body lies hid (for scientists and those of the medical profession) a fuller comprehension of the laws of matter and the laws of health. *A Treatise on Cosmic Fire*, Alice Bailey.

The theory of the etheric body stems primarily from the Eastern esoteric teachings, in which the emphasis is placed upon the subtle nature of man. The oriental asserts that the objective physical body is but the outward manifestation of inner subjective energies.

This body, consisting of fine energy threads or lines of force and light, is the archetype upon which the dense physical form is built. It can best be described as a field of energy that underlies every cell and atom of the physical body, permeating and interpenetrating every part of it, and extending beyond to form a part of what is commonly called the health aura. The Bible speaks of it as the 'Golden Bowl'. To those with deeper vision it is often seen as a web or network animated with a golden light.

This etheric framework consists of material drawn from the four ethers, which is built into a specific form. The network of fine tubular threadlike channels, commonly known as the nadis, are related to the cerebro-spinal and sympathetic nervous systems. These channels, depending upon the quality of energy they carry, pass to certain areas of the body via the chakras, or centres of force within the etheric body.

The integral unit formed by the etheric and physical bodies is basically the most important vehicle of man, as it connects the physical world with the subtle worlds. Through it the five senses are able to function on the physical plane, and progressively it is able to register the impact of energies flowing to it from the higher realms.

Seven grades or sub-planes of physical matter form the physical-etheric unit. They may be tabulated as follows.

	First ether	
	Second ether	
	Third ether	Etheric body
Physical man	Fourth ether	
	Gaseous	
	Liquid	Physical body
	Dense	

These grades of matter should not be thought of as existing in separate layers, but as a homogenous force field containing a variety of high frequency energies, which are held in one cohesive unit under the direction of the soul.

Each of the four types of attenuated matter or ethers are peculiarly specialized according to the level upon which they are found. Dr. Guenther Wachsmuth, in his study of the etheric formative forces, lists the four ethers under the following headings: Warmth ether, Light ether, Chemical ether, Life ether.

Each ether is said to have its own form-building tendencies, and the following basic geometric shapes indicate the workings of these ethers.

These basic forms, expressed in nature, indicate the predominant etheric formative forces that are active. The structural shapes of the vegetable kingdom vividly portray this process, as do the organs of the human body. For example, we can see the chemical ether as the predominant force in shaping the half moon shapes of the heart valves, and the valves of the blood vessels. The leaves of the plants and trees and the shapes of crystals all illustrate the workings of the etheric formative forces. The flow of these etheric forces will be discussed in more detail in the chapters dealing with diagnosis and treatment of disease in the etheric body.

There is in the human body a symbol of the distinction between the higher etheric and lower physical levels. It is quite simply the diaphragm, which separates the upper cavity of the body, containing the organs concerned with activities analogous to those of a spiritual nature, from the viscera which are concerned with the more mundane but necessary pursuits of a material nature.

The etheric body has three basic functions, all closely

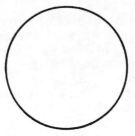

Warmth ether   Spherical forms

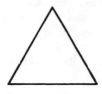

Light ether   Triangular forms

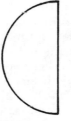

Chemical ether   Half moon forms

Life ether   Square forms

interrelated. It acts as a receiver of energies, an assimilator of energies and as a transmitter of energies. If each of these functions is maintained in a state of balance, then the physical body reflects this interchange of energies as a state of good health. The key to health lies in the correct reception, assimilation and distribution of energies. There are a number of factors which disturb the even circulation of energies throughout the etheric body, and these must be divided into two main categories — objective and subjective factors.

The objective factors are those within the substance of the etheric vehicle itself, preventing the even flow of energies to the various parts of the organism. They may be likened to large boulders jutting up from the bed of a stream, hindering the passage of the water as it returns to its source. Such obstacles either dam up the water, creating congestion, or the water flow is increased as it forces its way by.

These objective blockages are miasms, toxins, physical anomalies and diseased or traumatized areas. The miasms and toxins are perhaps the most dangerous elements to be considered, as their presence in the etheric substance undermines health in a most insidious way, often leading to gross organic pathology. Miasms may be classified under three major headings: syphilitic, tubercular and cancerous. They may be acquired during the lifetime of the individual, or hereditary. When a human being incarnates, it is said that he draws the material for his etheric body from the etheric vehicle of the earth, and the substance for his dense physical body comes from the earth itself. This matter, polluted by countless diseased bodies over millions of years, carries within it the seeds of the three major diseases. As the individual appropriates materials for his bodies, he may, if his present experience calls for it, acquire those elements which predispose him to certain disease patterns.

It is hard to put a clear definition to the word 'miasm', but it may be thought of as a paraphysical disease pattern, residing on etheric levels, in varying degrees of intensity and activity. This pattern is inevitably found upon the fourth or life ether. Its presence alone, undermines health. If the life of the individual transgresses the natural laws, then to that degree the miasm may be activated. Bad falls or emotional shock frequently precipitate the miasmic pattern from the fourth ether, so that it brings about gross pathological changes. How often we see in the case history of a patient, that their health deteriorated following a fall or other type of shock.

Toxins, like miasms, hinder the flow of energies through the etheric body. Such toxins may be of a bacterial or chemical nature. Childhood diseases leave toxic residue patterns which may upset the individual's health for years to come. Drugs leave their residues, as do chemical poisons which pollute our food and general environment. All of these disturb the function of the etheric body, and their removal is essential to optimum health.

There is a deep esoteric relationship between the etheric body and the kidneys. Both are concerned with reception, assimilation and transmission of energies, the kidneys expressing the more physical aspect of these processes. I believe it is significant that kidney diseases are on the increase, as this reflects the tremendous stresses that our etheric bodies are under, in this modern civilization.

Congestion of the etheric body is a major cause of disease. This congestion may be objective, that is miasmic or toxic, or it may be due to subjective factors found in the chakras or centres of force within the etheric body. Where there is an incorrect flow of energy through a chakra, congestion can occur, and this may be found in the etheric or astral bodies.

Overstimulation of the etheric body and its chakras is another prime source of disease, and the causes must always be sought out and corrected if health is to be reinstated.

Lack of co-ordination between the etheric body and the physical body can bring about poor health. This is frequently the case in trance mediumship wherein the etheric body is easily drawn out of the physical, in order to let a discarnate entity utilize the dense vehicle. Epilepsy, debilitation, impotence, obsession and laryngitis express varying degrees of poor co-ordination between the physical and etheric bodies. These matters will be dealt with in more detail further on in the book.

In summarizing, it suffices to state that the etheric body is the instrument of life which produces and sustains the physical form. It is the true intermediary or unseen link between the physical world and the subjective realms of the astral and mental levels. Upon its correct reception and distribution of energies, depends the health of the physical body. As radionic practitioners we should note that it is a potent receiver of impressions, which are conveyed to the consciousness via the chakras.

CHAPTER THREE

THE FORCE CENTRES

The importance of the seven plexii in any system of medicine, eastern or western, has still not been recognised or appreciated. It is indeed regrettable.

Gem Therapy, Dr. B. Bhattacharya

Having outlined the basic picture of the etheric body, it is now possible to enlarge upon it by giving a more detailed description of the chakras or force centres that occur in certain areas of the etheric vehicle. These chakras are of vital importance to the practitioner, because they are the focal points which receive energies for the purpose of vitalizing the physical body. It is through these centres that the healing energies are directed towards the diseased areas of the body, in order to bring about a state of equilibrium or health.

The force centres or chakras are located upon the surface of the etheric body, and appear as rotating vortices of subtle matter. Each centre is composed of three concentric, interblending whorls of energy, the rotations of which are speeded up and intensified commensurate with the inner development of the individual, until the chakra becomes fourth dimensional and capable of receiving and transmitting energy in a harmonious manner.

A chakra may be defined as a focal point for the reception and transmission of energies. These energies can originate from a variety of sources, some cosmic, others from the collective unconscious of a nation or humanity at large, or from the physical, emotional and mental worlds of the lower self. All make their impact upon the unit of human consciousness we call man, galvanizing him into action and determining his moods and characteristics.

The chakras in the etheric body come into being where the strands of energy cross and re-cross each other. The seven major chakras form where these lines cross each other twenty-one times. The minor chakras, of which there are twenty-one, occur where the energy strands cross fourteen times. Where the lines of energy cross seven times, lesser focal points are created, and there are said to be forty-nine such points. Beyond this there are many tiny force centres, which probably correspond to the acupuncture points of Chinese medicine.

The chakras have three main functions.

First   To vitalize the physical body.

Second   To bring about the development of self consciousness.

Third   To transmit spiritual energy in order to bring the individual into a state of spiritual being.

These centres are in the nature of distributing agencies, providing dynamic force and qualitative energy to the man. They produce definite effects upon his outward physical appearance, and through their continuous activity his character tendencies emerge.

It is important for the radionic practitioner to have a clear understanding of energy flow, as related to the function of the force centres. He should never forget that ENERGY FOLLOWS THOUGHT, and that a clearly visualized picture of the route taken by the healing energies, to their destination via the chakras, to the organ systems of the body, will in the final analysis increase the benefic action of his work.

The incoming energy, which is designated as the primary energy, and may be a healing rate, a colour or a homoeopathic potency radionically broadcast, enters the chakra situated in the etheric body. It is transmuted at this point by a process of differentiation into the secondary energies of the primary energy involved. This occurs automatically, the speed of the transformation and effect upon the physical body being determined by the condition of the chakra.

Having passed through the centre, the secondary energies play upon the nadis, causing the nervous system to respond, and in so doing pass the impulse on to the endocrine gland associated with the chakra. This effects a release of its hormones into the bloodstream, thus conditioning man and making him what he is at any given time.

Much of the ill health we see today can be traced directly to the condition of the chakras, as they determine the proper functioning of the aforementioned systems. Perfect co-ordination of the nadis, nerves and endocrine glands results in freedom from disease. Most of the early Westernized literature concerned with the chakras pays very little attention to their relationship with the endocrine sytem, and the affect of that relationship upon the health of the individual. This important factor cannot be overlooked if we are to gain a clear and practical picture of the etheric mechanism.

Basically the centre therapist is concerned with energy flow and distribution. It is his task to diagnose the imbalances that occur in the reception, assimilation and distribution of energies as they enter and circulate throughout the etheric body. The normal flow of energy entering a chakra and flowing unimpeded to its destination is illustrated on page 27.

The chakras in the etheric body are to be found in various states of activity. They reflect the physical, emotional, mental and spiritual quality of the individual, and may be found in any one of the following conditions represented by the five symbols.

The Circle: The chakra is simply a saucer-like depression, closed and inert, or rotating very slowly. There is no real intensity in its action, and the energy within it is just perceptible as a dim glow. The symbol further stands for the human body viewed from an etheric point of view. It symbolizes the single cell within the human body, or the atom of the physicist.

The circle with the point in the centre: The chakra is opening with signs of pulsation. It has a glowing point of energy in the middle of the saucer-like depression, and its rotation is becoming more rapid.

The circle divided into two: Here the activity of the chakra is quickening and alive. The point of energy at the centre is extending outward towards the periphery, it burns more brightly and due to its rotary action casts off energy in two directions, thus creating the appearance of a divided circle. The depression is becoming a vortex of energy, more brilliantly lit.

The circle divided into four: This represents the chakra which is radiantly active and seeking to blend with other chakras. Not only is the circle rotating but the cross within it rotates as well, creating an effect of great beauty. It indicates a high point of inner development, and is the true circle of matter, the equal armed cross of the Holy Spirit.

The swastika: Indicates that the point of energy at the centre of the chakra has extended to the periphery and is circulating around the periphery. This fiery wheel signifies the highest activity of matter, blazing and radiant throughout. Such a chakra becomes fourth dimensional and is better described as a sphere than a wheel. It is functioning in perfect unison with the other chakras.

During the course of making a diagnosis it will be found that each chakra of the patient falls into one of the first four categories. Because of these imbalances, due to the inability at this time to exert proper control over the energies flowing through the human form, disease and suffering become manifest.

In the Master Jesus all seven major chakras were perfectly balanced, correctly awakened and energized, making him an expression of perfected man. This is the example and promise that he held out to us, that each may become as perfect as him, and ultimately express the Divine Purpose.

Determining the condition of each major chakra is the main work .of the centre therapist. These force centres must be working properly in order to supply the physical body with

Incoming Primary Energy

Chakra

Outgoing Secondary Energies

Nadis

Nervous System

Endocrine System

Blood

the right amount and quality of energy. Any deviation from normal creates an imbalance which may ultimately lead to organic pathology.

Chakras can be damaged by traumatic accidents, and especially by sudden, dramatic, emotional shocks. Nagging fears or anxiety can, through constant wearing activity, disturb the functional balance. Chakras are frequently found to be blocked, either at the point where energy enters, or at the point where it exits to flow into the etheric body. If a blockage occurs at the entrance, the energy flowing in is frequently driven back to its point of origin on the astral or mental planes. This brings about psychological problems and endocrine dysfunction. If the blockage is at the exit, the energy builds up until enough pressure enables it to burst through to stimulate the appropriate endocrine gland. This causes erratic endocrine function with attendant physical and psychological problems. These blockages are of a subjective nature, as opposed to the objective nature of the blockages caused by miasms or toxins.

The following diagram illustrates the position of the seven major chakras, their glandular correspondences and the areas of the physical body directly governed by them. It should always be remembered that each chakra, although only present in subtle matter, externalizes itself on the physical plane as an endocrine gland, just as the nadis materialize as the nervous system. There are some texts which stress very strongly that the physical nerve plexii and endocrine glands should not be confused with the chakras. It is true that they should not be confused with the centres; on the other hand it is not correct to divorce the endocrine system from the chakras, as the latter are simply an extension of the former. It cannot be too strongly stated that the subtle anatomy directly relates to the physical. Acting as though they were separate factors only leads to a distorted view of the total man.

This diagram differs from the traditional Westernized concept of the chakra positions, with the exceptions of the crown and ajna centres in the head. Instead of placing the five other chakras over the front of the body, it locates them at approximately one inch above the dorsal surface of the

The Seven Major Spinal Chakras

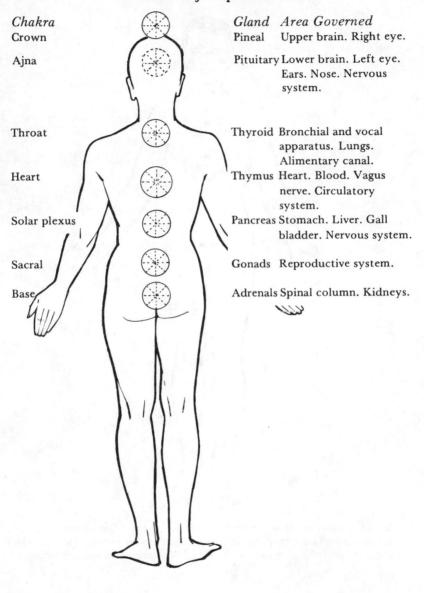

Chakra	Gland	Area Governed
Crown	Pineal	Upper brain. Right eye.
Ajna	Pituitary	Lower brain. Left eye. Ears. Nose. Nervous system.
Throat	Thyroid	Bronchial and vocal apparatus. Lungs. Alimentary canal.
Heart	Thymus	Heart. Blood. Vagus nerve. Circulatory system.
Solar plexus	Pancreas	Stomach. Liver. Gall bladder. Nervous system.
Sacral	Gonads	Reproductive system.
Base	Adrenals	Spinal column. Kidneys.

The Twenty-one Minor Chakras

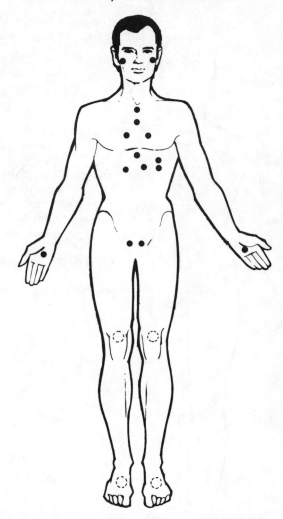

The locations of these minor chakras in the illustration are only approximate. Those marked with solid lines are on the anterior aspect of the body, and those shown with dotted lines are on the posterior aspect.

physical body, along the spinal column.

Due to the work done by astral psychics, we are accustomed to seeing the chakras positioned on the front of the body. This has occurred because astral psychics tend to work with certain involutionary energies. Thus through the illusion engendered by their inability to 'see' clearly, they place the chakras on the front of the torso instead of along the evolutionary path of the spinal column.

There is another inaccuracy often seen in Western writings on the chakras, showing the spleen chakra as one of the major centres. This chakra, although of vital importance, is not counted as one of the major centres. Earlier authors, having included it, found it necessary to omit one of the other chakras in order to keep the number at seven. They left out the sacral chakra and attributed its action of vitalizing the reproductive system to the centre at the base of the spine, which, as we have seen, governs the kidneys and spinal column. This compound inaccuracy prevents a clear, practical picture of the centres from being formulated, and naturally offsets the efficacy of any treatment that is designed to bring balance to the forces operating within the etheric body and its chakras.

As previously mentioned there are twenty-one minor chakras. These centres are, in the average and advanced person, governed by the action of the major chakras, and are treated via the nearest major force centre. However in cases where the major chakra is normally inactive, it may be necessary to treat the minor chakras directly. They are to be found in the following locations: one in front of each ear, one above each breast, one where the clavicles meet, one in the palm of each hand, one on the sole of each foot, one just behind each eye, one related to each gonad, one near the liver, one connected with the stomach, two superimposed, connected with spleen, one behind each knee, one near the thymus gland, one near the solar plexus.

CHAPTER FOUR

THE SEVEN MAJOR SPINAL CHAKRAS

> And I saw in the right hand of him that sat on the throne a book written within and on the back side, sealed with seven seals.
>
> *The Revelation of St. John*

Literally translated, the word 'chakra' means 'wheel'. It expresses the focalization or multi-concentric manifestation of the dynamic life principle in space. Ancient Eastern texts speak of the universe as a gigantic mandala, containing many other mandalas, or concentric force fields.

In the human body, the chakras or psychic centres signify the spatial unfoldment of the macrocosmic universal power on the level of the microcosm, thus bearing out the truth of the ancient Hermetic axiom, 'As above, so below'.

The ordered descent of the soul through successive gradations of subtle and physical matter provides a remarkable picture of the workings of Nature and the continuity of relationships between the subtle and physical anatomy. Let us trace this descent.

The soul upon incarnating draws to it enough of the universal chitta or mind stuff to form the mental body. Next, the less refined matter of the astral plane is used to form the emotional vehicle. Following this, the etheric structure is built from matter more coarse than that of the astral or mental planes. The subtle nervous system of the nadis is built from matter of the etheric levels, and this web gives rise to the physical nervous sytem. The next step down brings about the formation of the endocrine system. I do not suggest that each vehicle is built in that order, but that it represents a progression of appropriation of matter by the soul. Now we can consider the concentric centres of force in the etheric body, and their relationship to this progression.

Logically one would expect to find a chakra that projects a profound neural-endocrine influence. A chakra that supports all of the other centres, and relates to the preservation of the projected physical form, one that will guard the body on the physical plane. Such a centre is the base chakra.

The Base or Muladhara Chakra

This vitally important chakra is situated at the apex of the sacrum. Its primary externalization is the adrenal glands. It governs, as we can see from the chart in the preceding chapter, the kidneys and the spinal column.

The adrenals, which are the physical counterpart of the base chakra, are made up of an inner medulla covered by a layer known as the cortex. The adrenal medulla, consisting of chromaffine tissue, so named because of its affinity for chromium in laboratory tests, is in fact an endocrine extension of the autonomic nervous system that controls many body functions automatically.

Apart from the medullary tissue, there is spread throughout the body extra-medullary chromaffine tissue. This tissue arises in the embryo as neuroblasts. These primitive nerve cells migrate along the course of the sympathetic nerves, and are found in special concentrations along the sympathetic nerve chains running along each side of the spine, rather reminiscent of the ida and pingala nadis of the Vedic texts. They are also found in all of the major nerve plexii of the body, and are widely distributed throughout the dermis of the skin.

The adrenal medulla produces the hormone known as adrenalin. This secretion is responsible for readying the body for fight or flight in times of stress, thus preserving the physical organism from threatened damage or extinction. The extra-medullary chromaffine also produces adrenalin, so this protective system pervades the entire body, reinforcing the action of the nervous system and intensifying its activity.

It is interesting to see how clearly modern physiology comes to confirming what the ancient seers of India wrote many thousands of years ago. They observed that the base chakra was responsible for anchoring the body on the physical plane, and for providing a channel for the will-to-be to express itself. We know today that adrenalectomy is soon followed by death. May it not be because the link between the base chakra and the physical body has been severed by removal of the adrenals, and the will-to-be can no longer find a channel of expression?

They further observed that the base chakra animates the substance or cellular matrix of the physical body, feeding and directing the life principle, and underlying all other chakras. That certainly tallies with the fact that extra-medullary chromaffine tissue is found distributed throughout the body, with particular concentrations in the major nerve plexuses which are but reflections of the spinal chakras.

There is a large amount of chromaffine tissue on the ventral surface of the aorta, which appears so consistently that it is called the organ of Zuckerland. It is no coincidence that in this region, near the kidneys, appear two minor chakras related to the astral levels. These chakras let in much of the fear that people experience today, so nature has naturally placed them where glandular response can deal with the unwelcome incoming energies.

The base chakra is said to be relatively dormant in the mass of humanity, but its activity is on the increase due to the stress of modern living.

Premature over-stimulation can result in the burning away of the protective etheric webs along the spine, thus opening up the chakras to forces that the individual is not yet capable of handling. From this excessive stimulation, nervous instability and insanity may very easily occur. Our mental homes are filled with people who, for one reason or another, have lost to some degree the insulation provided by nature to protect them from certain aspects of the astral world and from the tremendous power of various cosmic forces. Those who foolishly spend time trying to open up the chakras by meditating upon them or stimulating them by other means, or by attempting to arouse the kundalini in an effort to take a spiritual short cut which does not in reality exist, are courting danger.

Unleashing of this incredible force along the spinal channels may burn everything in its path, including the permanent atoms. H.P. Blavatsky refers to such people as lost souls, because the ability to incarnate or function consciously on the lower planes is lost for aeons of time. The devastating effects of the prematurely aroused kundalini energy are well expressed in a recent book called *Kundalini – The Evolutionary Energy in Man* by Gopi Krishna. This autobiography points out the dangers and horrifying aspects of this experience.

Fortunately most people who dabble with this more glamorous realm of Yoga are protected by their gross ignorance of the subject, and an inherent inability to practise Yoga properly. However the radionic practitioner may have patients come to him who are suffering from overstimulation of the chakras, so it is essential to become familiar with the symptoms that arise from such imbalances.

The substance of the physical body is animated, as previously mentioned, by the base chakra. The kundalini energies, when correctly awakened and controlled in full consciousness, progress up the spine in a geometric pattern similar to the intertwined snakes of the caduces, symbol of the healing arts. Curiously enough the same pattern is also seen in the double-helix configuration of the DNA molecules, containing the code of life. Perhaps this too reflects a connection between the base chakra and the cellular substance of the physical body.

The miasms or inherited patterns of disease which are passed from generation to generation, or drawn in with the etheric substance during the process of incarnating, may be carried over from either source in the etheric template of the double-helix This may explain why any miasm can be dissipated and finally eliminated from the etheric body by treating the base chakra with colour. Toxins from chemical or bacterial sources respond in a similar manner, and it is a simple matter to clear them by the use of colour radionically broadcast.

Because it governs the spine, the base chakra is the focal point for treatment of any problems pertaining to the spine. Similarly kidney problems are treated by way of the base chakra. Psychological problems, where the will to live is at a low ebb, are treated via the base chakra and a series of other related centres. This technique will be dealt with in a later chapter dealing with treatment.

Base Chakra and Some Autonomic Nerve Plexuses

Each nerve plexus contains considerable concentrations of chromaffin tissue, thus indicating the connection of the base chakras to all other chakras.

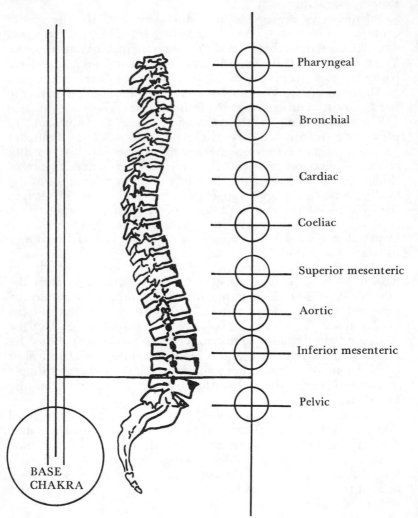

Distribution of Chromaffine Tissue and Base Chakra

Showing adreno-medullary and extra-medullary distribution along the sympathetic nerve chains.

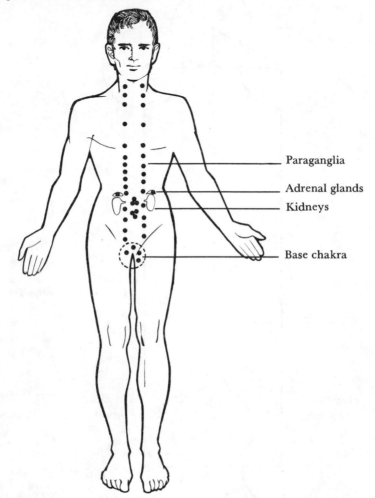

Paraganglia

Adrenal glands

Kidneys

Base chakra

Chromaffine tissue is also extensively distributed in the dermis of the skin.

Base Chakra and the Three Major Nadis
The Path of Life

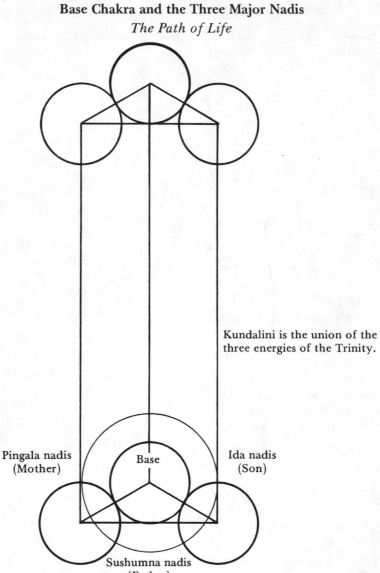

Kundalini is the union of the three energies of the Trinity.

Pingala nadis
(Mother)

Base

Ida nadis
(Son)

Sushumna nadis
(Father)

The preceding three illustrations deal with the base chakra and its relationship to the nervous system, the endocrine system and the kundalini energy which lies coiled at the base of the spine.

The Sacral or Svadhisthana Chakra

The sacral chakra is located at the base of the lumbar spine. It externalizes as the gonads, and governs the entire reproductive system. The degree of its activity is extensive and serves to guarantee the continuity of the human species.

Intense activity of this chakra will produce diseases of the reproductive system which are familiar to orthodox medicine and psychologists. Mystics, often successful in bringing in energies from external sources or from higher chakras, frequently overstimulate this centre. This is reflected in the sexual implications of Biblical writings which refer to the marriage in heaven, the bride of Christ and so forth. Inner energy transferences are used to sublimate sexual drives, but the terminology used reflects their origin.

Often in the course of mystical experience, which may cover several incarnations, there occurs a period of sexual imbalance. The mystic, in touching the higher energies, finds that they go straight to the sacral chakra instead of being expressed through the throat chakra which is the higher creative centre. This leads to stimulation of sexual activity and imagination, eventually leading to pathology both physical and psychological in nature.

Treatment of diseases found in the reproductive system is normally applied to the sacral chakra, however there are times when it becomes necessary to treat the throat chakra instead. This technique is designed to stimulate the action of the throat chakra, in such a way as to draw the energies up from the sacral centre, thus allowing nature to restore a balance in those areas governed by it.

The Solar Plexus or Manipura Chakra

The solar plexus chakra is located on the spine below the level of the shoulder blades. Its counterpart in the glandular system is the pancreas. This gland has both an exocrine and an endocrine function, the bulk of the gland secretes pancreatic juice, the enzymes of which help with the digestion of proteins, carbohydrates and fats. The endocrine part of the gland is formed by small clumps of cells called the islets of Langerhans, these secrete insulin which plays an important role in the control of sugar metabolism. The stomach is considered to be a secondary externalization of the solar plexus chakra.

Through this centre in the astral and etheric bodies, we find that humanity is conditioned by desire, be it good, bad, selfish or spiritual. This chakra is the vast clearing house for all of the energies found below the diaphragm. In the majority of people it is overstimulated, resulting in nervous disorders, stomach, gall bladder and liver diseases. It is frequently found to be overactive when radionically analysed.

Dysfunction of the solar plexus chakra is said to be one of the most potent causes of cancer. Certain reactions between this centre and the heart chakra cause congestion of the solar plexus centre. Energies connected with the life principle which is anchored in the heart, fail to find outward expression on the physical plane. This has a profound effect upon the bloodstream and brings about a proliferation of tissue, creating growths and tumours of a malignant nature. It is usual to find in such cases that the solar plexus chakra has a reading of minus or underactivity. In any case where a negative reading is found in connection with this centre, care must be taken to determine the presence of cancer, either as a miasm or as organic pathology.

Over-stimulation of the solar plexus chakra is connected with many kinds of skin eruptions, and leads to astralism, delusions, hallucinations and a wide variety of nervous disorders.

In order to quieten the action of this centre in the cases where it is overactive, colour and the use of Bach Remedies prove very effective. Where the reading is negative, first try to determine the presence of cancer or a pre-cancerous condition. If present it must be treated via the base chakra. Then the solar plexus chakra must be normalized so that it reacts properly to the energies of the heart, and most important of all the cause of the negativity in the solar plexus must be found, and steps taken to eliminate it. Usually it is of a psychological nature.

The Heart or Anhata Chakra

The heart chakra is situated between the shoulder blades, and its physical counterpart in the glandular system is the thymus. This gland, long recognized by the ancient seers as an endocrine secreting tissue, has now tentatively been included under this category in modern medical texts.

The thymus is described as being involved in hyperimmune or autoimmune reactions, and could prove important in such diseases as systemic lupus erythematosus, rheumatoid arthritis, ulcerative colitis and myasthenia gravis.

Certain experiments indicate that it helps in responses of the adrenal cortex to stress. The ancients would certainly agree to this, for they stated long ago that the thread of the life principle is anchored in the heart chakra and it would certainly be involved in the fight or flight mechanism designed to protect the expression of life on the physical plane.

The thymus is proportionately larger in the infant, and like the pineal and adrenal glands which are also connected with the will to express life on the physical plane, it undergoes involutionary changes.

When the heart chakra is overactive it produces the amoral, irresponsible individual. At present the full functioning of this centre is unsafe due to man's point of inner development, which is reflected in the general imbalance of the average endocrine system. Energy flooding uncontrolled through this chakra would have devastating effects upon the personality of the person concerned.

If correctly awakened, this chakra has transforming, magnetic and radiatory powers. Through it the 'Love of God is shed abroad'. It is said that the thymus holds the key to much that concerns the control and activity of the vagus nerve.

The raising of the energies from the solar plexus chakra up into the heart centre, occurs in those individuals who are developing the ability to think and act in terms of group consciousness, for example businessmen who preside over large companies. This transfer frequently throws great strain upon the heart centre with the result that many executives succumb to heart trouble. Doctors too are prone to overstimulation as they unconsciously seek to work through the heart centre in detaching themselves from the emotional aspects of the cases they treat.

Overstimulation due to working in group consciousness will result in heart problems. Overstimulation based on selfish motives may produce ulceration of the stomach, as the energies below the diaphragm are not drawn upward through the heart centre by the magnetic pull of unselfish motive. This is a matter which should be checked carefully in all cases where business executives or doctors seek radionic treatment.

All diseases of the heart, the circulatory system and the blood may be treated effectively via the heart chakra, utilizing colour and the appropriate remedies.

The Throat or Vishuddha Chakra

The throat chakra is located at the back of the neck, reaching up into the medulla oblongata to involve the carotid gland, and downwards in the direction of the shoulder blades. It is a powerful chakra and very active in the human family, being related directly to the higher creative faculties.

It manifests as the thyroid gland, with secondary expression as the parathyroid glands. These endocrine glands are essential to normal growth, the thyroid being related to oxidative processes and the parathyroids with calcium metabolism. If underactive, the throat chakra will cause a multitude of symptoms involving many tissues of the body.

Vertigo, allergies, anaemia, fatigue, menstrual irregularities, sore throats, laryngitis, asthma and other respiratory troubles may stem from an imbalance in this chakra. The damage resulting from sudden emotional shock will often initiate asthmatic states. This is understandable, because the throat centre governs the lungs, bronchial and vocal apparatus. It also governs the entire alimentary canal.

It is a centre which is peculiarly responsive to radionic treatment utilizing the colour blue, especially in its deep, clear shades.

The Brow or Ajna Chakra

This centre is located between the eyebrows, just above the eyes. It externalizes as the pituitary gland which lies within the small cavity formed by the sella turcica of the sphenoid bone. The anterior and posterior lobes of the pituitary gland correspond to the double multiple petals of the ajna chakra.

The ancient teachers considered the ajna chakra to be the centre of the integrated personality, and attached great importance to its role of expressing the fully developed personality of the individual. Modern medicine recognizes the pituitary as the master controlling gland of the endocrine system. It manages the activities of the thyroid, parathyroid, gonads, adrenals and pancreas.

These glands are referred to as target glands, and whenever they are producing the correct amount of hormone secretions the pituitary is at rest and therefore controlled by secretions from the other glands. Whenever a target gland fails to produce its correct quota of hormones, the pituitary goes into action and secretes a tropic hormone which, by way of the bloodstream, reaches the target gland and stimulates it into activity. If a gland is constantly underactive then the pituitary has to work overtime to try and galvanize it into activity. This creates an imbalance in the ajna chakra, making it overactive. So, in any case where the ajna reads as overactive, always search to see if the cause lies in another chakra which is underactive.

This centre is often referred to as the third eye. However this is just another inaccuracy that has crept into our knowledge of the chakras, a point that I will deal with in a later chapter. The anja expresses idealism, imagination and desire, and is rapidly becoming active in the masses of humanity. This chakra when active will exemplify itself in the typical hereditary pituitary type patient, who is usually attractive and magnetic in nature, has many irons in the fire and excels in business, with an enthusiastic capacity for leadership.

Overstimulation of this chakra can produce serious diseases of the brain and eyes, nose and ears and nervous system, which are those areas of the body which are governed by the ajna.

Sinus problems, catarrh and hayfever can all be traced to ajna imbalance. Gigantism and acromegaly also arise from deep-seated aberration of this chakra.

The Crown or Sahasrara Chakra

The crown chakra, as the name suggests, is located at the very top of the head, and is said not to come into full functioning until a high degree of inner development has been reached. Its dense physical externalization is the pineal gland, which when viewed from an esoteric point of view is seen to remain active during infancy, and until the will-to-be sufficiently anchors the child on to the physical plane.

It is interesting to note that Rudolph Steiner links this with the change of teeth at about the seventh year. Physiologists have little to offer regarding the pineal, except that its structure suggests an endocrine function, and that at the seventh year the human pineal undergoes an involutionary change and apparently ceases to function, thus providing us with a parallel to Steiner's observation.

The Greeks suggested that the pineal was the seat of the soul, which agrees with the ancient Indian esoteric tradition. Galen felt that it was connected with the regulation of thought. Recent experiments have shown that the pineal reacts to the stimulation from light, which ties in with Descartes' suggestion that there was a pineal connection between visual perception and evoked muscular response. The pineal gland contains vestigial retinal tissue and is considered by modern physiologists to have the possible function of a third photoreceptor, which all points to the pineal as being the third eye rather than the ajna centre.

The crown chakra governs the upper brain and the right eye. It is relatively inactive in the mass of humanity. Unfoldment of this centre brings with it hypertension, certain forms of brain disease, nervous disorders and various psychological problems.

The crown centre contains within it a replica of each chakra, thus it is a reflection of Brahman the macrocosmic principle, and at the same time it contains within its periphery the pattern of total man. Average and advanced man works through all of his chakras, but the highly advanced initiate increasingly works through the counterparts in the crown chakra, all his life focus being tuned in to the ultimate reality of the macrocosm. His energies so to speak function only from the throne of consciousness, and from this seat the inner man has access to the universe of cells, chakras and subtle vehicles, in order to express soul consciousness on the lower planes. One may liken the crown chakra to a master control panel which processes information flowing in from the external environmental fields, and outward from the inner spiritual realms. In modern terms it is the data processing computer utilized by the initiate to relay cosmic principles of truth to the lower planes of existence, analysing their effects and relaying this information back to the soul which has its seat in the crown chakra.

Full development of this chakra creates a vast aura of light, the beauty and magnitude of which eclipses every other chakra, and indicates the blossoming of perfected man, a god incarnate. The impulse towards physical incarnation ceases to exist and the individual evolves from the human kingdom into the spiritual kingdom. John speaks of this in the *Revelation* when he says, 'He goeth out no more.'

The ancient seers long ago recognized the importance of the pineal and thymus glands as externalizations of the crown and heart chakras. They taught that the Life principle was anchored in the heart by a thread of energy, and that the Consciousness principle was anchored in the pineal centre in a similar manner.

This cord of energies links the physical bodies to the subtle mechanisms. The thread linked to the head is disconnected when we sleep and physical consciousness leaves us, thus man enacts on a minor scale the process of life and death. The consciousness thread is temporarily severed during epileptic seizures and other forms of fainting, a point that the radionic practitioner should keep in mind when handling such cases. As long as the thread of Life energy remains anchored in the heart chakra the physical body will function. Coma occurs from a severe disruption of the consciousness thread. Death results from the severing of the Life thread. The Bible speaks of these combined energies as the Silver Cord which is loosed at death, thus freeing the inner man from the confines of the physical body.

As a chakra becomes active so its secretions and their effects can be observed. It is interesting that endocrinologists are at last grudgingly admitting that the pineal and thymus have an endocrine function, thus indicating that these chakras are becoming more active in the mass of humanity. We can expect to hear much more about them in the future, especially the pineal's relationship to light, for as the light of the soul begins to pour through this chakra, so will new discoveries be made, discoveries with far-reaching implications for man and all kingdoms in nature.

Just as seven major chakras are to be found in the etheric body, they are also seen in the astral and mental bodies, with the exception of the head centres, the throat and the heart which appear to be contained within the lotus of the soul upon the higher mental plane. Buckminster Fuller speaks of man as a multi-concentric halo system. This concept at once both ancient and modern can be illustrated in the following manner.

What a vast difference there is between this anatomical chart and the orthodox texts we habitually use for ordinary radionic practice. It expresses the concept of man as a series of energy fields, not a complicated mass of cellular structures and organic systems. It shows clearly the relationship of each force field and its chakras, and above all it is simple and practical.

Simplicity and effectiveness should be the guide to every practitioner's approach to radionics, and this can never become a reality as long as we are dealing with man from the physical to the subtle. It is essential to think of man first as a series of force field systems, and that pathology begins there before appearing in the physical body. It isn't enough to talk of the etheric heart or the etheric lungs, this is still thinking in physical terms. What the practitioner must do is to recognize that the chakras are the source of power that determine the physical, mental and emotional makeup of the individual, and as such they are the key to his health and well-being. To ignore this fact is to use a fragmentary approach to radionics, and our

Man Radiating Outward from the Solar Lotus
of the Soul

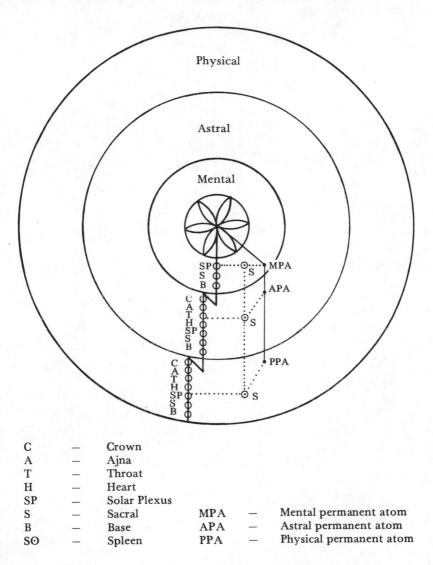

C	—	Crown			
A	—	Ajna			
T	—	Throat			
H	—	Heart			
SP	—	Solar Plexus			
S	—	Sacral	MPA	—	Mental permanent atom
B	—	Base	APA	—	Astral permanent atom
S☉	—	Spleen	PPA	—	Physical permanent atom

one aim is to treat the total man. This can only be done in the light of an understanding of the chakras and their relationship to all bodies, dense or subtle.

CHAPTER FIVE

VITALITY AND THE DYNAMICS OF PRANIC RECEPTION

By a comprehension of the laws of vitality — and in this phrase are comprehended the laws governing prana, radiation and magnetism — will come the healing of the diseases in the blood, of the arteries and veins, of certain nervous complaints, lack of vitality, senile decay, poor circulation and similar ills.

Esoteric Healing, Alice Bailey

In this chapter I am going to deal with the very important topic of vitality. One of the most frequent complaints we hear from patients is that they are chronically tired. Clinical evidence suggests that providing patients live sensibly, radionic treatment can do much to improve their vitality, thus enhancing their ability to throw off disease.

Vitality is closely linked to the correct functioning of the spleen chakra, so it is necessary in any diagnosis of the chakras to determine the condition of this centre. Prana or vital force is distributed from the spleen chakra to all of the other major chakras, and from there sent to the organic systems of the physical body.

'Prana' is a Sanskrit term, which broadly translated means 'life-energy'. It is the life essence which works through the four ethers, and manifests in the activity of matter; without prana there would be no physical manifestation. This form of energy is responsible for maintaining the integrity of the physical-etheric vehicle. Its presence in correct proportions is essential to health, and it is for this reason that the radionic practitioner must give it careful consideration.

There are various types of prana, but our main concern is with that form of prana which emanates from the sun. Solar prana radiates through our entire solar system, and is assimilated by all forms, be they planetary, human, animal or vegetable. Each form absorbs this prana, circulates it, and keeps what is required to maintain its integrity. The excess, now saturated with the distinctive qualities of the form it has passed through, is discharged back into the etheric force field of the earth to be utilized by other forms of life.

To these individual qualified pranic emanations are given the names, planetary prana, human prana and so forth. In the etheric field of the solar system there is a continual exchange of pranic currents between the various planets. On the microcosmic level the human etheric vehicle assimilates a mixture of solar and planetary prana, and then discharges the qualified excess back into the etheric body of the earth, to mix with the prana found therein. The plant and animal kingdoms function in a similar manner, so that a vast interchange of energies can be seen to go on, using the etheric web as a medium for transmission.

It is the human prana which manifests as the health aura. When being discharged this blends with the pranic excess radiating from the atoms of the dense physical body, and produces an area of radiation that is commonly mistaken for the etheric body.

The health of the etheric body, and hence the dense physical, depends upon prana, and the healing arts are moving towards a recognition of this fact. For example it is now understood that sunlight plays an important part in the building up and maintaining of health. By virtue of this fact sanatoria are often placed in the countryside, close to the sea, or on mountain slopes where the air is clear and heavily charged with the life-giving prana. In such conditions patients are able to rebuild their depleted systems far more rapidly than in the contaminated environs of our cities.

The growing recognition of the importance of vitamin therapy in the treatment of various diseases is another indication of man's growing awareness of the vital forces in nature, and the part they play in restoring health. Science now recognizes that vitamins and their synergists are essential to the normal physiological processes of the body, and that a total lack of a single vitamin in the diet, say vitamin C or one of the B complex can eventually result in the death of the organism.

If we consider this in the light of what has already been written, it is evident that vitamins, as the name suggests, do in fact supply pranic vitality to the vital or etheric body.

In some quarters it is strongly upheld that man obtains enough of the vitamins he needs from his everyday diet, and perhaps in the past he was able to do so. Today however, with an increasing array of devitalized foods on the market, many of which are saturated with preservatives and other toxins that have an insidious effect in undermining health — and the fact that moderm man lives under tremendous economic and psychological pressures — the role of vitamins in supplementing the diet needs careful consideration on the part of the radionic practitioner.

Another point of consideration relative to prana, is the fact that in recent years the practice of yoga has become popular in the Occident, and people are doing breathing exercises designed to increase their intake of prana.

These exercises, known as pranayama, are aimed at cleansing the body of impurities and filling it with pranic currents, thus increasing vitality and instilling a feeling of well-being. It should be pointed out, however, that many of these exercises, if practised with diligence, can be very dangerous to Western man and may bring about overstimulation of the etheric body with subsequent psychic and physiological disturbances.

Frequently the type of patient who asks a radionic practitioner for help will be one who is familiar with such exercises, and may in fact practise them. For this reason it should be kept in mind that pranayama incorrectly practised may be a root cause for etheric dysfunction.

Pantanjali, the Indian philospher, lists five differentiations of prana in the human body. The healing rates of these pranic forces are very useful to the practitioner who consciously works on the etheric levels, and they may be directed through the appropriate chakras to the areas concerned. The list is as follows.

1. *Prana,* extending from the nose to the heart, and having special relation to the mouth and speech, the heart and lungs.

2. *Samana,* which extends from the heart to the solar plexus. It concerns food and the nourishing of the body through

the medium of food and drink, and has a special relation to the stomach.
3. *Apana*, which controls from the solar plexus to the soles of the feet. It concerns the organs of elimination, of rejection and of birth, thus having special relation to the organs of regeneration, and of elimination.
4. *Upana*, which is found between the nose and the top of the head, and has a special relation to the brain, the nose and the eyes.
5. *Vyana*, which is the term applied to the sum total of prana in the human body.

The implications inherent in these differentiations of prana and radionic therapeutic measures, are self evident. For example in cases of hayfever or chronic sinus trouble, treatment of the ajna chakra with upana and the required colour is going to be significantly useful. The rate for samana directed via the solar plexus chakra will help a patient to absorb nutrients more fully, and the rate for apana directed by way of the sacral chakra may prove most useful in treating a patient during childbirth, as supplementary to regular medical care.

Certain manifestations of prana may be observed directly by the human eye. Atoms that have become heavily charged with prana manifest as brilliant white dots of light that dart and spin through the atmosphere. It is especially easy to see them on a clear sunny day against a blue sky, by simply focusing the eyes at a distance of about six feet and observing them move through the intervening space in a silent erratic dance. The esotericist gives to this energy dot the name of vitality globule; such particles of matter are being continually taken up by the etheric body, so that they can play their role in vitalizing it.

Dr. Wilhelm Reich, who did much experimentation with the pranic energies, or orgone energy as he preferred to call it, came to the same conclusion as the Indian sages. He said, in effect, that there was a primordial, universally present energy, and that this energy penetrated and permeated everything, manifesting in the living creature as biological energy, and in the universe as the origin of galactic systems, matter and movement.

Pranas and the Human Body

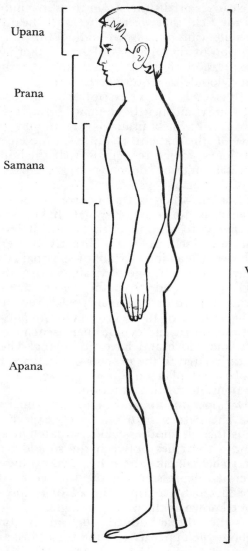

Upana

Prana

Samana

Vyana

Apana

He further stated that the earth, people, animals and plants are all surrounded by individual orgone envelopes which can be seen quite clearly, and distinct from the surrounding orgone ocean. This is the field that we refer to as the health aura, the coarsest of visible vibrations surrounding the human form. Reich's description of the orgone dot as a flickering, spinning and darting expression of the universal energy, tallies exactly with the vitality globule of esoteric literature.

Having briefly sketched in a description of the pranic forces and their role in vitalizing the human form, we can now consider the way in which prana is taken into the etheric body. Vitality of the patient is always of concern to the radionic practitioner, for he recognizes that the body's ability to restore normal function depends in great part upon the vitality levels of the various systems.

The spleen chakra which is that centre of force so closely related to vitality, is not a major spinal chakra. Its role is to supply vital energy to all the chakras on all levels of the personality or lower self. It is not directly related to those energies which sweep man into a state of spirituality by way of the major centres. Its role is one of vitalizing the etheric body.

It must be understood that the seven major chakras appeared during the course of man's early evolution, as a response to the impact of the seven major streams of energy that are said to comprise the evolutionary scheme of things in which we live and move and have our being. They are not however directly related to the process of vitalizing the etheric body with solar and planetary prana, a separate group of chakras are responsible for this function.

The receptive apparatus for prana consists primarily of three force centres. The best known one is the spleen chakra; in addition to this there is another chakra situated just below the diaphragm, and a third lies between the shoulder blades just above the heart chakra. Like the other chakras they appear as rotating saucer-like depressions in the surface of the etheric body, and are linked by a triple thread of energy to form a triangle of force known as the pranic triangle.

Prana enters the etheric body through minor force centres found throughout the upper part of the torso. It is then drawn down to the spleen chakra, and enters to circulate through the triangle formed by the three chakras. Before being discharged from the spleen centre to vitalize the etheric body, the prana is subjected to a process that regulates its potency.

If the organism is a healthy one, the vibratory rate will be stepped up. If the health of the individual is poor, then the rate of potency will be stepped down, so that the vitalizing effect of the prana will not disrupt the etheric body.

Assimilation takes place after the prana has been circulated through the triangle of force set up by the three pranic chakras. It permeates the etheric web and creates a state of vitality in accordance with the ability of the organism to receive prana. Thus the dense physical body and the etheric vehicle are maintained in one cohesive unit, and will remain so until the silver cord is loosed, and contact with the etheric body is broken, resulting in death and finally disintegration of the earthly vehicle.

From the orthodox point of view the distinctive function of the spleen remains unknown. To the student of subtle anatomy it provides an interesting correspondence to the placenta and the umbilical cord, which connects the foetus to the mother for nutritional purposes. This cord, as we well know, is cut when the birth of the child is complete. Similarly the etheric silver cord is cut when the physical and etheric bodies are separated at death, and the inner man is 'born' in full consciousness, into the world of a higher and more subtle dimension.

In assessing the vitality index of a patient, the radionic practitioner must determine whether the pranic energies are being received, assimilated and distributed properly by way of the spleen chakra. The other two centres in this pranic triangle should also receive attention, particularly the one between the shoulder blades, as it is profoundly affected by distortions or subluxations of the dorsal spine, tensions in the upper and mid-dorsal musculature and general poor posture. All of these factors disturb pranic circulation and utilization and ultimately lead to a state of fatigue.

It is significant that Dr. Abrams almost always percussed the spinous process of the seventh cervical vertebra in order to

The Pranic Triangle

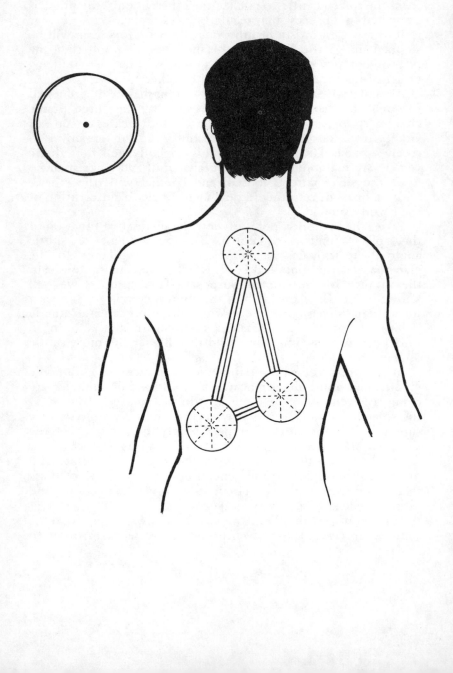

dilate the spleen. He fixed this dilation by percussing the spinous of the second dorsal vertebra. Then he was ready to begin radionic treatment of his patient. .

Abrams said that by dilating the spleen, toxic factors and the miasmic poisons were drawn into the spleen. Localizing them in this manner he was able to clear them from the patient in short order; by painting the necessary medicine over the spleen and applying the treatment pads to the area, he got an additional response.

Although Abrams had a sound physiological basis for percussing the spinous processes of the cervical and dorsal vertebra, the centre therapist would tend to see a deeper implication in his action, namely that by dilating the spleen he was in effect stimulating the action of the spleen chakra for a short period, and that this carried the subtle energies of the remedy painted on the body, throughout the etheric vehicle and in fact to all of the major spinal centres. Naturally this would have a profound healing effect upon the body.

If, as radionic practitioners, we understand the nature of vitalization of the human form by solar energies, we are going to be in a better position to help our patients. Sir Thomas Browne once wrote, 'Life is a pure flame and we live by an invisible sun within us.' This thought may be interpreted in various ways according to the level about which you are speaking, but on the physical-etheric it certainly refers to the spleen and its action of receiving the pranic forces from the sun.

CHAPTER SIX

THE CENTRE THERAPY INSTRUMENT

The whole world surrounds man as a circle surrounds one point — And wisdom, whether it be heavenly or earthly, can be achieved only through the attractive force of the centre and the circle.

Paracelsus

Before going into the practical aspects of diagnosis and treatment of the subtle anatomy of man, it is necessary to touch briefly upon the subject of radionic instrumentation in the light of what has been written so far.

Early on in my investigations into radionics, I was struck by the fact that all of the instruments that were presently available, and the techniques for their use, were simply modifications on the same theme. Although the etheric aspects of matter were recognized in radionic circles, there was no evidence to suggest that they had been used as a point of departure in the development of new radionic instrumentation, or to create better techniques of diagnosis and treatment. As far as I could determine no real departure had been made from the legacy of the physically orientated approach, left to us by the early pioneers in this field.

I felt that if a radionic instrument is to be used on etheric levels, and that is surely where all radionic instruments function, then it would be better to build an instrument that, by its very layout and functional qualities, keyed itself to the etheric levels. If an instrument and the techniques for its use relate directly to the laws and actions of the etheric formative forces, then one may assume that such an instrument would prove more effective in its action, the benefit ultimately accruing to the patient. So I decided to attempt to build an instrument that would meet these specifications.

In theory the project was very interesting to anticipate, but my initial enthusiasm was severely put to the test when I realized that the numerous layouts that I was designing had too many similarities to existing sets. No matter how much I worked at it, it appeared impossible to make a break from the old concept of instrument layout. After several months I finally gave up the project, and decided to make do with the instrument I had.

At this point a curious thing happened. No sooner had I given up the idea of creating a different kind of radionic instrument, than the answer I had been seeking for so long suddenly presented itself quite intuitively. It was this. *Apply an organic geometric form to the dial placing, one that is relative to the chakras and the etheric formative forces.*

The circle was obviously the only answer, as it did in fact reflect an etheric principle to be found in both micro and macrocosm. The chakras are themselves formed by three concentric circles of energy, and the flow of the etheric formative forces is also, as we shall see, related to the circle.

Encouraged by this insight I began to read through two volumes on etheric geometry by George Adams, hoping to find some evidence to support the idea of circular dial placing. For my part I knew with absolute conviction that the idea was correct, but it would be interesting to see what agreement might be found in the writings of those individuals with a profound knowledge of the etheric formative forces. For anyone wishing to study the principles of etheric geometry in order to relate this knowledge to radionics, the two books *Physical and Ethereal Spaces* and *Space and The Light of The Creation* by Adams are both highly recommended.

In the books by Adams I found that Rudolph Steiner is quoted as having written the following statement relevant to the basic action of the etheric formative forces: 'The etheric formative forces pour centripetally inward from the circumference of cosmic space.'

Adams himself had written, 'The circle manifests the isotropic property of metric space — equal units of measure in all directions.'

Looking further afield, I read through Wachsmuth's *Etheric Formative Forces in Cosmos, Earth and Man*, and found the following statement: 'The circle encloses all the colours and forces in the spectrum of light and of Nature — the world of spiritual being flows into the world of substance.'

Paracelsus obviously felt that the circle was a very important symbol and frequently referred to it in his writings. I found this reflection upon it. 'Everything that man accomplishes or does, that he teaches or wants to learn, must have its right proportion; it must follow its own line and remain within its circle, to the end that balance be preserved, that there be no crooked thing, that nothing exceed the circle.'

In *Ideas and Integrities*, the autobiography of the American architect Buckminster Fuller, I found yet another reference to the circle, and what must be one of the most interesting summaries of the workings of the etheric formative forces to come from a modern source. He writes:

> The circling bands of a cross-sectioned tree or the scalloped terraces of the shell fish are convergently secreted structures (intereferences of a higher order) of cyclic bundling of experiences. Wave embodiments of cyclic experience appear everywhere in the accredited morphology of nature's omni-directional, convergent-divergent, synchronous-dyssynchronous, infinite plurality of pulsating controls of interactive events in principle. The cyclic wave accretions — unique to parent and parent's parent — make overlapping internal impressions of the periodic and cyclic inter-ferences-structuring-by-accretion, prearranging thereby internal angles of original turbining tendency of unfoldment, upon the gestating seed of periodic secretion of outside-in and then inside-out pulsation-inversion, which we call regenerative birth. This is, of course, a union of the infinite inwardness with the infinite outwardness to fulfill the comprehensive duality of uni-verse. Human egos are multi-concentric halo systems.

Here Fuller speaks of a human being as a multi-concentric force field, and his conclusion coincides with the ancient seers who stated that three circles were symbolic of the lower self of man, and of the chakras to be found therein.

Having decided to use the circle as a form for the dial positioning in the new instrument, as opposed to the straight line layout of other sets, I gathered my thoughts on the subject together and wrote them in my note book under the following heading.

Geometric Dial Placing

In order to ensure a full relationship between the flow of

the etheric formative forces and the radionic instrument, the dial placings must conform to the circular periphery of cosmic space. Thus there is less resistance to the reception and distribution of energies.

The dials or resonators are placed geometrically in circles in order to act as *selective coupling units*, linking the peripheral, centripetally flowing etheric formative forces to the earth form of the sample plate and patient witness. This creates a harmonic relationship between the instrument and the hypothetical infinite periphery of space, that will conjure inward, through rate selection, those energies that will offset the lack of harmony within the patient.

Circular rate setting acts as an invocative centre of force. The patient is related harmonically through the circular spacing of selective coupling units, to the cosmic periphery, thus the attracted energies can seek to bring equilibrium to the imbalance within the patient's frequency systems.

It is a verifiable fact that the energy field within a frame or pattern is automatically intensified. One has only to look at an unframed painting and then frame it, to see the action of the frame upon the vitality of the painting. The circular linking of the selective coupling units, and the inscribed pattern of the instrument panel itself, provide a frame of considerable potency in which the patient sample is placed.

From these notes and ideas the Mark I Centre Instrument was developed. It was a large instrument with three circles of resonators. The inner circle carried treatment rates, the middle circle the chakra to which they were being directed, and the outer circle carried the rate for the gland or organ relative to the chakra being treated. In this way a flow of treatment was represented. The circles were also used in another way. The mental body rate was put up on the small inner circle for diagnostic purposes, the middle row was used for the astral diagnosis and the etheric on the outer circle. The instrument turned out to be remarkably sensitive, but rather large for convenient use.

Next to be developed was the Mark II, a much smaller instrument' using only one circle of dials. This set was electrically powered and contained a five watt light source to

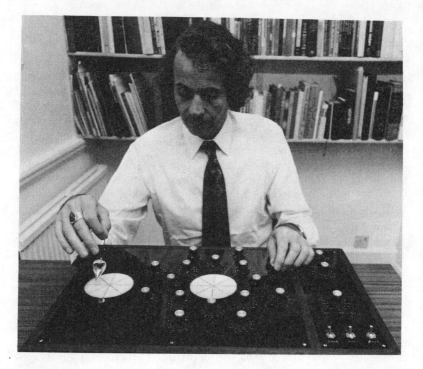

project colour across the resonators and patient sample inside the instrument. It also utilized a small speaker which set up vibrations at right angles to the colour flow, and directly towards the blood spot. It was limited in as much as only one rate could be put up, representing a chakra or one of the subtle bodies into which the colour was placed. Once again it proved to be very effective for broadcast treatment, so I set out to design and build a set which was a compromise between the Mark I and the Mark II.

Further work produced the Mark III Centre Instrument, which appears in the illustration. It consists of two panels in a mahogany box with a divider between them. The panel on the right contains the sample and detector chambers, both rotate freely for correct positioning during diagnosis and treatment. Each is carrying a pattern specific to the operator who uses the instrument. This does not mean that another individual would not be able to work the box, but that it is designed to work at maximum sensitivity for the owner. Much is made of the individuality of radionic practitioners and their approach to radionics, so it seemed logical to produce sets for individuals rather than on a predetermined design.

The sample plate is surrounded by two circles of dials, and the detector plate over which the pendulum is used sits on the right. The sample plate is slotted to allow the blood spot or hair sample to be placed inside the instrument. The small panel on the left is the control panel. This contains three switches at the top for mains electricity, light and sound. The knob below the switches enables the operator to modulate the intensity of the light beam for treatment.

Next, there are holes drilled to contain ampules of homoeopathic medicines, and in front of them is a slot in which colour transparencies are placed for chakra treatment. The next knob is a measuring dial marked from 0 to 100. This is used, as the name suggests, to measure the intensity of imbalances in the various chakras or subtle bodies. Below is another knob surrounded by the five symbols described in chapter three. These are used to determine the state of evolvement of each chakra. The entire instrument measures about 22 inches by 14 inches, so is fairly compact and easy to work with.

The light source which carries the medicine or colour frequencies over the resonators in the large section of the box, sits directly behind the colour slot in the middle of the small panel. A speaker is positioned below the sample chamber, and is used to vibrate a diamond pattern which respresents the pattern of the planetary etheric web. Speakers are used extensively in India to vibrate precious and semi-precious stones for teletherapy purposes, and I have found that they work effectively in conjunction with the visible colour spectrum.

The circular placing of resonators or selective coupling units brings with it a unique factor, which to date has not been considered in the field of radionic diagnosis or treatment. By using a circular arrangement of dials one has the advantage of being able to bring the selected rate into a critical rotational position relative to the centripetal flow of the etheric formative forces and the patient sample. Some reflection on the part of the reader will reveal the advantages of being able to rotate the rate.

In keeping with the purpose of its design, that is to key itself to the etheric levels, the Mark III utilizes the following. Electricity, which has its initial vibration on the plane of the first ether. Light, which has a close connection with, and uses as a medium, the second ether. Sound, which functions through the third ether, and is the ether of numbers too; and colour, which is allied to the fourth ether. So each ether that is to be found in the human etheric body is represented in the set.

Having created an instrument, the next point to consider was the numerical values for the rate dials. There has been much speculation concerning the significance of numbers, but it is reasonably safe to say that the real inner secrets of this science died with Pythagoras.

George Adams had written that the circle manifested the isotropic properties of metric space. This was little indication that ten would be a suitable number to use, but it did offer a possibility. Supporting this possibility was the fact that the ancient teachings venerated the number ten as the greatest of all numbers because it comprehends all arithmetic and harmonic proportions and is the nature of number itself.

Relative to the circle and number I found the following in Adams' book on etheric geometry. 'Now as we pass to the flower, and from the hidden plastic principle there emerges more or less suddenly and evidently a manifest property of Number. In the characteristic circular form of the flower, we see a great variety of cyclic number pictures, mathematical in nature.' And: 'Over against the blossom of the plant there is the human blood in the circulation of which a hidden music of number is likewise at work.'

Upon this apparently tenuous link of metric space, the circle and the number pictures in the circular forms of blossoms and blood circulation, I decided to use the number ten as the rate value for my Mark III instrument. Abrams, Ruth Drown and George de la Warr had all calibrated their instruments from 0 to 10, and I could find no reason for using a different number.

There are two circles of dials on the instrument, eight resonators making up each circle. All rates used on the instrument consist of eight digits. This was an arbitrary choice but it had a comfortably encompassing organic feeling about it. Subsequently I was to find that eight is considered to be the number of regeneration. Ten as harmony and eight as regeneration seemed ideal qualities to use in a radionic set.

I believe that using the circle or circular shapes in the design of any instrument connected with the absorption and distribution of energies may find extensive use in other fields of experimentation. For example in America the Bell Telephone Company has developed a lead acid battery on these principles. It is said to have a life span of thirty years, and the remarkable thing is that this battery becomes stronger and more efficient the older it gets. Probably the circular placing of the lead elements inside attracts energy and stores it in rather the same manner as an orgone accumulator.

Certainly the employment of circular dial placing in the radionic instrument has a great advantage over standard layouts. By utilizing a natural principle of the flow of the etheric formative forces, both diagnosis and treatment reflect a simplicity and accuracy that can be had in no other way.

CHAPTER SEVEN

DIAGNOSIS AND THE SUBTLE BODIES

The new medical science will be outstandingly built upon the science of the centres, and upon this knowledge all diagnosis and possible cure will be based.

Esoteric Healing Alice A. Bailey

Even to the layman, if he stops to think about it, the human form presents an amazing complexity and variety of parts. There are billions of cells, each performing a role aimed at integrating the diversity of structures into a smoothly functioning organism. Each part dependent upon another for its existence. Stop the heart and the whole organism fails; destroy certain brain cells and a part falls useless or the personality of the individual is radically altered.

All of these functions and processes are revealing their secrets to the march of medical science, so that today there is an ever growing mass of information about men as a highly complex and co-ordinated series of organ systems. In contrast there is little to be found in the scientific texts about man as a force field system.

In 1935 Northrop and Burr put forward their electro-dynamic theory of life. This revolutionary concept of life as force field systems, while not immediately accepted with open arms by the more orthodox scientists of the day, has subsequently proved to be one of the greatest steps forward in the study of life from the angle of energies and force fields.

Radionics, if it is to progress, must move towards a recognition of man not simply as an electro-magnetic force field but as something more. Science has taken up the work of investigating life from this point of view, and naturally the workers in this field will do a thorough job. As science spends more time investigating the energy fields of life it will confirm the early work of radionic pioneers, and will be able to accept the basic concepts of this method of diagnosis and healing.

However, the spearhead of any investigation radionically

carried out must always be ahead of the prevailing thought of the day. For this reason the next step ahead for radionics is the development of diagnostic techniques based on the subtle force fields of man. Not the electro-magnetic fields but the etheric force field with its centres of dynamic force that feed and maintain the physical organism.

Regular radionic diagnostic procedure is a long and detailed process, something entailing protracted periods of tiring work, which frequently leave the practitioner drained of energy. These physically orientated methods, dealing as they do with the organic systems, cannot in the final analysis arrive at the cause of disease. It is essential to determine the conditions existing in the force centres and the subtle bodies, in order to get near to the cause of imbalances in the human force fields.

The technique of diagnosis as utilized by the centre therapist is directed straight at the etheric body with its seven major force centres. This phases out the irrelevancy of the billions of cells which make up the physical form with its organic systems, and concentrates upon the energy field that activates them. It must ever be kept in mind that the physical body is simply an automaton, the life processes of which depend upon the activity of the underlying force fields which we call the etheric, astral and mental bodies.

The diagnostic procedure in centre therapy is quite basic and simple in conception. It determines the condition and activity of each major chakra and the spleen centre. The state of the etheric body and the presence of miasms or toxins in that vehicle. This then is the first phase.

The patient sample, be it a blood spot, lock of hair or saliva sample, is placed in the sample chamber of the instrument, and rotated into the critical rotational position as indicated by the action of the pendulum over the detector plate. The detector plate is then rotated into a critical position relative to the sample, thus giving the correct juxtaposition of the geometric patterns of each chamber for the purposes of the diagnosis.

Next the IRP or individual rate pattern of the patient is determined. This is done by turning each dial until a reaction is noted; the number indicated is then written down. This is repeated with eight dials until the full rate for the patient is obtained. It may read as follows, 77538024, and represents the patient as a whole. This number remains on the outer circle of dials until the diagnosis is completed. The IRP is employed rather than a symptom rate because it contains the picture of the entire patient, and not a fractional factor such as a symptom.

Having done this the diagnosis can proceed. First the vitality index of the patient is determined by mentally asking for the vitality level of the patient, and measuring it off on the measuring dial. This is noted on the case sheet, 75 to 80 being normal for most operators. Then the spleen chakra is checked to see if it is overactive, underactive or normally active, because the state of this chakra has a direct bearing on the vitality of the patient. If the spleen chakra is under or overactive, it should be checked for blockages at the entry or exit points. If a blockage is found it should be entered on the case sheet. Next check the condition of the other two pranic force centres in a similar manner, and enter any findings that may occur.

Having ascertained the condition of the pranic centres and the vitality index of the patient, attention can be turned to the seven major spinal chakras. The procedure for their analysis is similar to that applied to the spleen centre.

Beginning at the crown chakra and working down to the base, each centre is checked in turn. The practitioner asks mentally if the crown chakra is overactive, underactive or normally active. According to the condition of the chakra, the case sheet is marked with the appropriate symbol, +, −, or N, each of which is self-explanatory. It should be understood that in seeking to determine the state of the chakra, the practitioner is not trying to determine a fleeting condition, but the absolute basic condition of that chakra. For example one may find a patient with a solar plexus chakra that gives a reading of underactive. A sudden fright would certainly bring about a great deal of solar plexus activity, but it would be temporary and not reflect the true state of the chakra. The basic state of a chakra does not change day by day, from one condition of activity to another, it remains steady and tends to change slowly under the impact of treatment or the alteration of character traits by the patient's own efforts.

Where there is a condition of over or underactivity, the degree of imbalance is measured off and noted. The progress of this reading towards zero following treatment may be used as an indication of progress towards normal balance of the chakra.

If the crown chakra reads + or — then it must be checked for blockages which may be present and causing the imbalance. With the degree of imbalance registered on the measuring dial, the practitioner mentally asks if the chakra is blocked. If a positive response is indicated by the pendulum, then it must be determined if the blockage exists at the point where energies flow into the chakra, or where they exit to make their impact upon the endocrine gland, in this case the pineal body. The following symbols are used to denote a blockage.

Entry blockage   0·
Exit blockage   ·0

Where a blockage is indicated, these symbols are entered upon the case sheet.

This procedure as outlined for determining the condition of the crown chakra, is then repeated for the ajna, throat, heart, solar plexus, sacral and base chakras, and the findings listed.

Having analysed the state of each chakra, the practitioner then turns his attention to the etheric body as a whole, and seeks out those factors which may be inhibiting the flow of energies throughout the etheric vehicle. First the presence of miasms must be accurately determined. There are quite a number of different labels for the miasms, but the centre therapist is concerned with the three major ones. These are syphilis, a disease which comes to mankind by courtesy of the Lemurian civilization, tuberculosis passed on by the Atlanteans, and cancer which is the disease of the present Aryan civilization.

It is interesting to note that both syphilis and tuberculosis have been brought under control, representing as they do the physical and emotional aspects of man's evolutionary development. But the permissiveness of today is releasing certain energies in various sections of society, with the result that the syphilitic expression of disease or energy imbalance is on the increase. For the most part, individuals in the present age are concerned with the development of their mental bodies. This activity carried forward consciously or unconsciously, with too much emotional suppression, produces cancerous conditions.

The miasms then are syphilitic, tubercular and cancerous. It is said that under these three headings all disease can be categorized. Patients may have one or more miasms in combination which undermine their health in general. Samuel Hahnemann, the founder of homoeopathy, listed the miasms as syphilitic, psora and sycosis. The reader is well advised to spend some time studying literature on the miasms, because these factors, if present in the etheric body, contribute much towards ill health, and their removal by homoeopathic or radionic means is essential to health.

Toxins from bacterial, chemical or drug sources may be sought out and noted. Personally I rarely bother with them now, as I have found that treatment of the chakras eliminates them anyhow, without them having been identified in detail. Miasms and toxins along with the intensity should be entered on the case sheet.

Next the overall condition of the etheric body is determined. Here three factors are of importance.
1. Congestion of the etheric body.
2. Overstimulation of the etheric body.
3. Lack of co-ordination.
    a. Between the physical and etheric bodies.
    b. Between the etheric and astral bodies.
If any of these conditions are identified, they should be measured for their intensity, and the appropriate notes made on the case sheet.

This concludes the diagnosis of the etheric body and its chakras. Treatment is determined upon these findings without any effort to look into the problems of the astral body. This is not to say that imbalances in the astral body can be ignored, they cannot, for the simple reason that they do cause much of the disease we see today.

However if we study the effect of treatment of the etheric

chakras, an interesting phenomenon comes to light. By removing blockages from the chakras and normalizing their activity, the practitioner releases the flow of energies in two directions. First the energies can flow freely into the etheric body, thus normalizing endocrine function. The effect of this is to bring a balance in the other direction, and the astral body becomes more harmonious in its action. Remember the chakras and endocrines which are the physical counterparts of the centres govern not only the physical appearance of an individual but also his personality traits. Normalization at that point affects physical and psychological factors in one approach.

Treatment of just the miasms or toxins in the etheric body is a very one-sided approach, and I speak of this from some experience in the use of techniques aimed at that end. Frequently patients who are treated in this manner may find very little difference in their health despite the face that certain miasms have been eradicated. The reason for this is simply because the chakras which supply energy to the etheric-physical body are not functioning correctly, and, until they are, ill health will be the lot of such a patient.

A striking example of this is treatment with endocrine extracts. Where a patient has a deficiency, this can be supplemented by oral administrations of the glandular extracts required, and health is restored in this manner. Withhold the gland extract and the patient will become ill and probably die in extreme cases of endocrine failure. As long as the chakra remains in a state of imbalance the endocrine gland associated with it will not function correctly. Dr. J. Samuels applied short wave treatment to endocrine glands in order to stimulate their function, and this proved more successful than oral administration of gland extracts. Once again however the cart is before the horse — endocrine glands only work as well as the chakra that governs them. Treatment aimed at bringing balance to the chakras has a more significant effect in the long run. One such approach is centre therapy.

If after one or two months' treatment of the etheric chakras, progress of the patient slows down, or perhaps has not gone along as well as expected, then it is time to check the astral body and its chakras. The procedure is exactly the same, each chakra is analysed, the astral body is then checked for factors such as fear, anxiety, depression and so forth, each psychological factor being checked and, when identified, noted down as to type and intensity.

The astral body is also checked for congestion, over-stimulation and a lack of co-ordination with the etheric or mental bodies. Overstimulation is a frequent cause of trouble to be looked for.

As for the mental body, I have never found the need to analyse its contents. Most disease originates on the emotional and etheric levels and for this reason our attention should be mainly focused on these levels.

There follows a sample case sheet showing an analysis of a patient's chakras and etheric body.

Accurate diagnosis of the centres is of course very important if the treatment is to be effective. More important however is the ability of the practitioner to interpret his findings. The key to correct interpretation of the information obtained from diagnosis of the chakras and the subtle bodies, lies in a knowledge of the centres and their relationship to the organic systems of the body.

It is the ability to interpret findings that makes a competent practitioner. Fortunately this ability cannot be imparted by way of the written word, it is something that must be drawn out of experience and through hard work, and the use of the intuitive mind. In this way what I have written in this book, and the technique I am describing, is protected. The dilettante will soon lose his way, and the serious student will forge on, building upon the basis which this book provides. What I am writing merely scratches the surface of the subject, and the ramifications can only come to light through expanded consciousness on the part of the practitioner.

Now to return to our case sheet and see what kind of interpretation can be put upon the findings. The patient is thirty-five years of age, with a history of sinus trouble and poor vitality, accompanied by digestive disorders, especially of the stomach. First his spleen chakra is functioning very poorly, and this would in part account for the lack of vitality. His

Centre Therapy Analysis Sheet

Name J. DOE		Age 35	Date 7.5.70

Address The Merton, La Canada Calif Tel:

Past Illnesses Suspected ulcer of Stomach. Catarrh

Present condition Debility - Sinusitus

Vitality Index 55·	Spleen Chakra 23 — 0.

CHAKRAS	+—N	BLOCKAGES	ASTRAL	MENTAL
Crown	N			
Ajna	57· —	·O		
Throat	40· +			
Heart	10· —			
Solar P.	N			
Sacral	N			
Base	N			

MIASMS — TOXINS — PHYSICAL ANOMALIES
Syphilitic miasm

	ETHERIC	ASTRAL	MENTAL
CONGESTION			
OVERSTIMULATION	✓		
LACK OF CO-ORD.			

NOTES

vitality index at 55 is too low for a man of his age.

Of the major chakras, three show an imbalance. The ajna is underactive, and this, because it governs the nasal area, will have a direct bearing on the sinus problem. The fact that it is both underactive and blocked will create a situation in which the individual will have difficulty in expressing himself as a personality. This can lead to unconscious feelings of self pity which frequently occur with sinus and catarrh conditions.

The block at the exit of the ajna is naturally going to create an endocrine imbalance, the pituitary is going to function erratically. Among other things the pituitary manages the function of the pancreas, so there is a link here between the stomach disorder and the ajna chakra.

The throat chakra is overactive, therefore the thyroid is going to be in a similar condition. The patient is burning up an excess of energy and yet the spleen being underactive is not really supplying anywhere near the amount needed. This indicates that the spleen chakra is going to need direct attention to stimulate its function.

The heart chakra is underactive, but not too badly. This may point out circulatory trouble and disturbed vagus function, an important point to consider, keeping in mind the profound effect this nerve has on body functions.

The etheric body contains a syphilitic miasm. This miasm tends to affect the throat (thus relating to the throat chakra problem), the eyes (bringing in the ajna chakra and the sinus area again), and the brain with its relationship to the vagus.

The etheric body shows a condition of overstimulation, energy is circulating too rapidly and is discharged before it has a chance to be absorbed and utilized . . . yet another factor in the fatigue problem. Usually the miasm is the cause for this condition of the etheric body. Remember a miasm can speed up or slow down the circulation of energies.

This briefly then is an interpretation of the preceding analysis of the chakras and the etheric body in relationship to the health of the person concerned. The analysis is simple, quick and gets right to the point, covering the main factors concerned, without going into endless details regarding the physical organic systems. Upon the basis of this analysis an effective programme of treatment can be quickly assessed, and I will follow this through in the next chapter so that a clear example is available for reference.

CHAPTER EIGHT

CENTRE THERAPY

By finding out the defective chakra and then correcting it with the appropriate cosmic ray, will be the key to the cure of such terrible diseases like T.B., cancer, insanity and epilepsy which are the despair of the doctor.

Magnet Dowsing, Dr. B. Bhattacharya

All forms of healing, irrespective of their origin, are directed towards one goal: the restoration of harmony and balance to the complexity of energies and matter that blend to form the subtle and physical anatomy of man.

The centre therapist differs from the orthodox radionic practitioner in as much as he utilizes the subtle force systems of man as his point of departure for diagnosis and treatment. The physical organic systems are of secondary importance, because they can only respond to and reflect the measure of harmony found in the paraphysical bodies. As previously mentioned, unless the chakras are functioning in a reasonably balanced and harmonious manner, there can never be an expression of health upon the physical level. Recognizing this, the practitioner aims his treatment specifically at those chakras which exhibit a state of imbalance. By normalizing their action and removing blockages, he enables the energies which are seeking expression through the low self to have free play, thus restoring health to the organism.

The prime healing agent used in centre therapy is colour. These colours are supplied through the use of cinemoid material which is mounted in 35mm film holders. These fit into the colour slot of the Mark III instrument, and light is used to carry the colour over the resonators and the patient sample located in the centre of the sample chamber. Colour has been found to be the most effective healing agent for this particular form of radionic therapy. Homoeopathic remedies in glass ampules and radionic healing rates are used to a much lesser degree. Colour is related to the fourth ether whereon most disease patterns of an etheric nature are located, perhaps for this reason it is most effective.

The procedure for determining treatment is as follows, each question being posited mentally.
1. Which of these chakras exhibiting an imbalance require treatment?
2. In what order should they be treated?
3. Which colours are required to normalize each chakra?
4. To which physical gland or organ should the colour be directed?
These questions based on our hypothetical case would produce the following treatment programme.

Violet ⟶ Spleen chakra ⟶ Etheric body
Orange ⟶ Heart chakra ⟶ Vagus nerve
Blue ⟶ Ajna chakra ⟶ Nose

There is no indication that the throat chakra requires treatment, and in fact the normalization of the ajna may directly influence this centre in the course of treatment.

The next factor to consider is the syphilitic miasm. The procedure is to ask which colour is required to disperse the miasm. Having determined for instance that it is green, the practitioner must then ascertain which gland or physical organ is to receive the beneficial effects of the green healing energy. As all miasms are treated by way of the base chakra, this leaves the choice of adrenals, kidneys or spinal column. The most frequent channel is the kidneys, which is perhaps to be expected as their job is to clear the body of certain waste products. So the treatment for this factor would read as follows.

Green ⟶ Base chakra ⟶ Kidneys

It can be taken as a rule that if the base chakra comes up for treatment because there is an imbalance in its action, then there is no need to select a colour to clear any miasms present. Practice shows that miasms disperse through the action of any colour placed into the base chakra. On the other hand if the base does not require treatment, then it will be necessary to find a colour to treat the miasm by way of that centre.

In order to set up a treatment the individual rate pattern is removed from the outer circle of dials. Taking the spleen for treatment in order to increase vitality, the violet slide is placed in the slot. Next the practitioner places his left index finger on the dial of the inner circle which is nearest to him, and then mentally asks if the rate should begin at this dial. This is repeated going around the circle in a clockwise direction until a positive response of the pendulum is obtained. Such a response indicates that the rate for the spleen chakra begins at this dial, and the rate of eight digits is put up on the instrument. The same procedure is repeated on the outer circle in order to find the starting point for the rate for the etheric body, to which the energy is to be distributed.

This technique for selecting the critical rotational position for the rates to be used during the treatment is unique to this type of instrument, and is found to be a distinct advantage over the straight line set up of conventional sets. In standard procedure the patient sample is rotated into a critical rotational position, but in centre therapy both the rates are put into their own CRP relative to not only the patient sample but also to the inflowing energies flowing from the hypothetical infinite periphery of space.

Some may wonder why the rate for the chakra is put up on the inner row of dials, and the gland, organ system or vehicle on the outer circle. The reason is this. The etheric formative forces stream inward until they reach a central point, then they return once again to the infinite periphery, thus a rhythmic flow of energies is set up. The etheric geometrician states that every point in space is at the centre of the universe, and that energies stream to and from that point ceaselessly.

For our purpose the centre of the sample chamber containing the patient sample is the central point to which the energies flow, and from there they are directed towards the patient. This is why the chakra rate is set up on the inner circle, because logically it receives the energy first as it flows from the central point on the return journey to the infinite periphery. The flow of energy in healing goes to the chakra and then to the gland or area governed by the chakra, and that is why the gland or organ rate goes on the outer circle. By setting up the treatment in this manner the proper sequence of events of the healing act are symbolized on the instrument.

Having got the treatment set up on the instrument, the mains, light and sonic switches are put on, thus activating the set. Next the intensity of light required for the treatment is determined by turning the light modulation dial until a positive response from the pendulum is obtained. The intensity of the light seems to have a direct bearing on the length of the treatment, the higher the intensity the shorter the treatment. It is perhaps significant that Dr. Iredell who treated terminal cancer patients at Guy's Hospital in London with colour, found that it was very important to be able to control the intensity of the light while treating these patients, and also that they responded much better if placed in a circular enclosure of black material during treatment. If the shape of the enclosure was varied, even without the patient knowing, they then complained that the treatment did not feel so strong.

Length of treatment depends no doubt on many factors, so this must be checked each time, simply by asking and watching for a positive response from the pendulum. There are so many variables that the practitioner must not be surprised if on one day a two minute treatment is indicated, and that on another fifteen minutes is required. Better to tailor the treatment length to patient demand than give them a set time each and every treatment.

The same flexibility must also apply to colour selection. There are no hard and fast rules that certain colours are used for treating certain chakras. Every individual has a different calibre of physical and etheric body. Chakras are vibrating at different speeds, and disease patterns are of an individual nature too. For this reason colours will vary for each patient, one may need green to clear a blockage in a chakra, whereas another patient with what appears to be an identical condition, needs violet or yellow.

There are of course certain broad generalities that may be applied to colours. For instance blue and green have a calming effect, and are found to be very useful in the treatment of acute conditions. Blue is usually excellent for low back pain, if placed by way of the base chakra to the spine. Green will have a calming effect for headaches if applied to the ajna chakra and nervous system. Green is a colour very frequently used to treat the ajna centre, and in India emerald gem medicines are used to treat conditions allied to the brow chakra. Blue seems to have an affinity for the throat centre and is very useful for treating conditions of the lungs such as asthma, or for sore throats and bronchial troubles.

Reds and oranges on the other hand are stimulating and may be used to increase vitality and tone up the circulatory system by way of the heart chakra. Varicosities may be treated in this manner. Yellow too is an excellent stimulant, especially for toning up the nervous system.

Violet is often used in infectious conditions as it tones up the etheric body, and helps it to throw off the vibratory force of the invading bacteria or virus. To augment the violet one may add an ampule of potentized onyx to the treatment. Onyx is said to carry the frequency of ultra-violet which is well known for its bactericidal qualities.

Each of the factors in the case which need treatment are taken in turn, and a card may be prepared showing which chakras and systems are to be treated. It is advisable to set this card on the instrument during treatment, not only for purposes of reference, but also to identify the blood spot's donor. In a busy practice it is all too easy to put a blood spot down and lose track of who it comes from. Naturally it is kept in a cellophane package, but for treatment it is removed and placed in the slot, so it is best accompanied by the treatment card.

The following guide to the effects of certain colours on the chakras, subtle bodies and miasms is included to provide the practitioner with some general information on the subject. It must be remembered that there are no hard and fast rules, colours for certain chakras or conditions will vary at times, and those set out here are the ones that seem to occur most frequently in practice.

The crown chakra is stimulated by orange, green, blue and indigo. It is calmed by red, yellow and violet. Indigo and violet are the best colours for removing blockages from this centre.

The ajna chakra is stimulated by red, orange, blue and violet, and calmed by yellow, green and indigo. The colour best suited to removing blockages is green.

The throat chakra is stimulated by red, and calmed by

orange, yellow, green, blue, indigo and violet. The best colours for removing blockages are blue and violet.

The heart chakra is stimulated by red, orange, indigo and violet. Calming effects can be obtained from yellow, green and blue. Red and indigo remove blockages from this chakra.

The solar plexus chakra is stimulated by red, orange, yellow, green and violet. Calmed by blue and indigo. Orange, yellow and blue remove blockages of the solar plexus chakra.

The sacral chakra is stimulated by red. Orange, yellow, green, blue, indigo and violet have a calming effect. For removal of blockages use blue or violet.

The base chakra is stimulated by green, indigo and violet. Red, orange, yellow and blue have a calming effect. Green is the supreme colour for removing blockages of this chakra.

The spleen chakra, supplier of pranic energies to all of the other chakras, is stimulated by red, orange, yellow, green and violet. Blue and indigo have a calming effect. Yellow, indigo and violet remove blockages of the spleen centre.

The practitioner will frequently detect miasms in the etheric body, normally located on the level of the fourth ether. As colour functions on this ether, miasms readily disperse when subjected to colour frequencies broadcast to the base chakra. The following colours are suitable for clearing the three basic miasms.

The syphilitic miasm clears through the use of yellow, green, blue or indigo.

The tubercular miasm should be treated with yellow or green.

The cancer miasm responds to red, green, blue, indigo and violet.

Conditions of the etheric body may require specific colours to normalize them, so for congestion use green, blue, indigo and violet. For overstimulation use green to obtain a calming effect. For lack of co-ordination between the physical and etheric vehicles, as occurs in petit-mal and other similar conditions, green is the colour of choice.

Astral problems are often found so it is as well to know the best colours for these factors on the astral level. For astral congestion use blue. Overstimulation calls for green or blue, and lack of co-ordination between the astral and etheric bodies is best treated with green.

For the mental body one finds that all conditions respond best to indigo.

Inflammation of the brain, certain brain tumours and some forms of insanity are treated via the crown chakra. The calming colours are selected in such cases in order to quieten the action of the crown centre which is usually overactive in these conditions.

Any problems related to the pituitary body are treated via the ajna chakra. Neuritis, migraine headaches, regular head-aches, eye and hearing problems as well as hayfever, sinus and catarrh trouble all respond to treatment of the ajna. Many disturbances of the nervous system may be treated via this centre as it governs the lower brain stem. Migraines are usually caused by a lack of balance between the force fields of the pineal and pituitary glands, so look to both of the head chakras when tackling this condition.

Heart trouble, certain diseases related to the autonomic nervous system and the vagus nerve, and circulatory trouble should all be treated via the heart chakra.

Diseases related to thyroid imbalance are treated by way of the throat chakra. Respiratory diseases such as asthma and tuberculosis, bronchitis and emphysema are all treated via the throat chakra.

Once in a while the practitioner may have a patient where the will to live is very weak, and the individual is at a very low ebb, not caring if he lives or dies. In such cases there is a definite procedure to follow. The will to live is expressed through two main chakras, the crown and the base. The crown is concerned with the will to be from a spiritual angle, and the base chakra is related to the will of the physical body to remain in incarnation. These energies expressing themselves as 'Persistence in Form' work through two triangles of force. The spiritual aspect works through the ajna, crown and throat chakras.

The practitioner must first determine which triangle of force must be treated in order to increase the will of the patient to remain in a physical body. It may be one of them, it may be

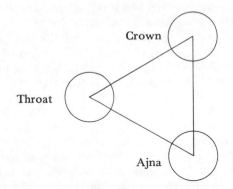

The lower expression concerning the physical form works through the following triangle of force.

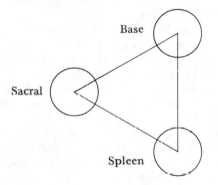

both. If both triangles are indicated for treatment, then determine in which order the treatment should run.

Having determined which triangle, select the colour required, and supplement it with the Bach remedies of Larch and Sweet Chestnut. If the lower triangle is treated, then begin with the base centre, then treat the sacral chakra and finally the spleen. Always follow this order and put the gland associated with the chakra being treated, up on the outer circle of the instrument dials. If the higher triangle requires treatment, then it is the crown which receives treatment first, then the throat and finally the ajna. If these treatments are set up on standard treatment sets instead of the Mark III centre therapy instrument, the rate for the chakra is followed by the appropriate endocrine gland. Colour transparencies and the Bach remedies are then placed on the plate along with the blood spot.

Nervous troubles, ulcers, diabetes, certain forms of cancer, gall bladder disease, liver trouble and digestive problems are best treated via the solar plexus chakra. Skin eruptions too are frequently treated through this centre. The solar plexus as a rule is overactive in the majority of people and should be treated with the appropriate colour to calm its action. If the practitioner obtains a negative response indicating that the solar plexus is underactive, it is well to seek carefully for a condition of cancer or a pre-cancerous state. Certainly if this negative solar plexus is found in conjunction with a cancer miasm, the patient is heading for cancer at some time in his or her life. This may be dispersed radionically or with the appropriate homoeopathic similimum.

Diseases of the reproductive system are all treated by way of the sacral chakra. In some cases however it is better to treat the throat chakra which is the higher creative counterpart. If such a measure is indicated then a colour to stimulate the action of the throat chakra should be selected. This form of treatment will draw the energies up from the overstimulated sacral chakra and enable it to return to normal.

Due to the stress and strain of modern living, back problems and so called slipped disc are increasing at an alarming rate. Stress of an emotional nature is not readily associated with back pain, but there is a direct relationship. Under stress, the adrenals which are governed by the base chakra pour adrenalin into the blood stream in order to cope with the problems (imagined or actual) at hand. Adrenalin contains certain constituents which inhibit the normal maintenance and upkeep of ligament tissue. The ligaments, especially those of the low back area, such as the ilio-lumbar and sacro-iliac ligaments, may stretch more than they should, especially if they have been damaged in the past. This stretching tears the sensory nerve fibres imbedded in the ligaments, this creates pain and the muscular system goes into a state of spasm in order to stabilize the affected area and give the ligament a chance to heal. This condition is often referred to as slipped disc, lumbago and even sciatica as the nerve pathways usually refer pain down the legs along one trajectory or another.

So all spinal problems and stress-created diseases should be treated via the base chakra. Kidney troubles are related to this centre too. The importance of treating this chakra in a wide variety of cases cannot be stressed too much. Ruth Drown placed great importance upon treatment of the adrenals in every abnormal condition. As mentioned previously, ALL miasms are treated through this centre.

Back problems in the cervical and upper dorsal spine may respond better if treated via the alta major chakra. This centre is located just at the base of the occiput and governs the spine. Its physical externalization is the carotid gland. This chakra has a direct relationship with the pituitary, base and heart chakras, being involved in the balance of tissue fluids and regulation of blood pressure.

The concept of treating the chakras radionically is only an extension of the work of Abrams and Ruth Drown; both of these pioneers utilized the endocrine system to improve their treatments. Abrams percussed the spinous processes of the seventh cervical and second dorsal vertebra to dilate the spleen, thus increasing the intake of vital force. Ruth Drown stated flatly that endocrinology was the very foundation of radionic diagnosis and treatment, and that the glands represent balance in the body, creating both mental and physical well-being.

Her opinion based on fact is certainly correct. The endocrine system governs our physical appearance and determines our emotional and mental characteristics. The centre therapist simply takes the concept one step further and states that the chakras govern the glands, therefore it is logical to treat the centres in order to bring harmony to the human form and its underlying force fields.

A most important factor to consider in treating the chakras is the proper use of visualization and thought. There is an ancient axiom that energy follows thought. It becomes very evident in practice that utilizing thought as the directing agency for the healing energies increases the efficacy of treatment. The power of this process is augmented by visualizing the healing energies flowing to the chakra being treated, and dispersing to the gland or organ system involved.

In this manner the imposition of a healing energy and pattern is placed upon the force of the disease, in order to disrupt its balance. Healing is accomplished by the use of correctly directed energy, and detailed visualization of the point of entry for that energy into the human force field system. As the healing energy leaves the chakra to circulate, it begins its work of stimulating every cell and atom, thus eliminating or palliating the disease condition present in the patient.

CHAPTER NINE

ETHERIALIZED MEDICINES

Diseases and their cures are nothing but Names and Forms, and
they have their origin and end in cosmic light.
Septenate Mixtures in Homoeopathy, B. Bhattacharya

Although colour is the principle therapeutic agent used in the
centre therapy technique for treating disease patterns found in
the subtle anatomy of man, there are times when homoeopathic remedies are found to be a useful adjunct to the colour
waveform.

Most homoeopathic remedies come from natural sources,
and approximately six hundred are in common usage. These
medicines are derived from the animal, vegetable and mineral
kingdoms, also from bacteria, insects, reptiles, snake venoms
and human sources. Their preparation is unique, using as it
does the techniques of dilution, trituration and succussion, to
produce remedies which, in the higher potencies, do not contain even one identifiable molecule of the original substance.

Apparently, this form of preparation releases what George
Adams refers to as the peripheral forces of the material, thus
enhancing its medicinal value and unveiling the healing spirit
within the substance. This release of energy from form, or
etherialization, makes homoeopathic remedies eminently suitable for treating the subtle vehicles of man, and restoring
harmony and balance to the forces operating within them.

The remedies used in centre therapy can be placed under
three headings: the Bach remedies, the gem remedies and the
regular homoeopathic medicines. First I will deal with the
Bach remedies.

During the six years following 1930, Dr. Edward Bach perfected a system of healing based, with one exception, upon the
use of flowers taken from the trees and plants of the countryside. The blooms were picked at specific times and, according
to the indications, medicines were prepared by floating them

in bowls of water and exposing them to sunlight, or by simply boiling the blooms in water. Spirit was then added to preserve the solution which resulted from these preparations.

Dr. Bach, like any true healer, was concerned with treating the organism as a whole. The diseases of the patients did not interest him as much as the moods or fears and anxieties that they exhibited. He felt that if these moods or fears could be dispelled, the organism would recover under the resultant influx of healing energies. In the light of esoteric knowledge it is easy to recognize the accuracy of this conclusion, reached by a man so sensitive as to be able to register the qualities of a flower by simply placing it upon his tongue. One is reminded of the great German mystic Jacob Boehme, demonstrating this same capacity to see into the heart of the plant kingdom.

The Bach remedies are specifically related to treatment of the emotions and states of mind to be found in man, therefore they make their impact directly upon the astral body, and, in some instances, upon the mental body. Such action naturally aids in bringing about healing on the etheric levels as well.

Most of our emotional states involve the solar plexus chakra. It is there that we feel the impacts of fear, anxiety and a host of other emotional feelings. In extreme fear the sacral and throat chakras become involved with the resultant loss of control of the urinary and anal sphincter muscles or temporary paralysis of the vocal chords. The Bach remedies without exception work through the solar plexus chakra, two of them directly involve other centres.

The following remedies make their impact upon the solar plexus chakra on the mental level.

Olive	Hornbeam
Gentian	Oak
Cerato	Cherry Plum
Willow	Agrimony
Scleranthus	Vine

The astral solar plexus is directly affected by the following Bach remedies. Two of them, Larch and Sweet Chestnut, are slightly different in their action. Both of course work through the astral solar plexus chakra, but Larch affects the throat chakra too, and Sweet Chestnut works through all of the astral body chakras.

Sweet Chestnut	Holly
Impatiens	Star of Bethlehem
Mimulus	Crab Apple
Centaury	Gorse
Walnut	Elm
Mustard	Larch
White Chestnut	Heather
Pine	Aspen
Red Chestnut	Rescue Remedy
Wild Rose	Water Violet
Beech	Rock Rose
Chestnut Bud	Clematis
Honeysuckle	Wild Oat
Vervain	

The remaining remedy Rock Water was found to work simply upon the etheric body, and once again through the solar plexus chakra.

In the booklet *The Twelve Healers*, Dr. Bach gave the indications for the use of Sweet Chestnut in these words: 'For those moments which happen to some people when the anguish is so great as to seem unbearable. When the mind or body feels as if it had borne to the uttermost limit of its endurance, and that now it must give way. When it seems there is nothing but destruction and annihilation left to face.'

Could it not be that when an individual is faced with what seems to be inescapable annihilation, it is necessary for the entire chakra system to be thrown into a positive state of activity, in order to counteract the negative polarity of the astral body under such circumstances? If so, then Sweet Chestnut would be the best Bach remedy for this purpose, for all the indications are that it is well suited to galvanize the astral body into positive activity.

Larch too is interesting in this respect. Here we have a remedy that works through the astral solar plexus, but also

affects the throat chakra. Dr. Bach gave the following indications for its use. 'For those who do not consider themselves as
good or capable as those around them, who expect failure,
who feel that they will never be a success, and so do not
venture or make a strong enough attempt to succeed.' People
who expect failure, or who do not have sufficient creative
drive to bring a project to a successful conclusion, naturally
require stimulation of the creative aspect of the higher nature.
If you recall that the throat chakra is the higher creative centre
in the human mechanism, and the counterpart of the sacral
chakra, this radionic conclusion that Larch works through
both the solar plexus and the throat centres is inclined to
make sense. Larch, then, works directly through the throat
chakra to bring out the best creative abilities in those who feel
that they are lacking in such qualities.

Bach remedies are often used by radionic practitioners, and
there can be no doubt as to their value in restoring health. It
should be borne in mind that any remedy that works on the
mental level will also be effective on the two lower planes, and
those which work on the astral will also affect the etheric
body. There is always greater healing power to a remedy that
works down from the higher levels to the lower, but as the
three bodies of the low self interpenetrate, remedies are never
totally confined in their effects to one vehicle. Thus mimulus,
for example, may well prove beneficial to the mental body but
does not work directly upon it.

Next for consideration are the gem remedies. These
medicines are made from various precious and semi-precious
stones, and are ideal for treating the chakras radionically
through broadcast techniques. Dr. A. Bhattacharya uses them
extensively at his clinic in Naihati, India. Many patients take
them orally, but up to two thousand patients are treated daily
with gem frequencies broadcast from the clinic's teletherapy
instruments. Results of these treatments at a distance bear
witness to the effectiveness of the healing powers of the gems.

Before dealing with each gem and its qualities, a word or
two about the preparation of these excellent medicines. Small,
good quality gems are purchased, and each is placed in a glass
vial containing a diluted alcohol solution. This is stood in dark-

ness for a week, allowing the vibratory force of the gem to permeate the solution. At the end of a week the gem is removed and washed in water, dried, and placed in storage for future use. Sugar pilules are then introduced into the solution and the vial rotated upwards and downwards gently until the pilules are well soaked in the radiated solution. They are then removed and dried on white paper, later to be stored in appropriately marked glass containers. These medicines can then be given orally when indicated. The gems last forever so the practitioner has the means to always make his own medicines as the need arises, without going into any complicated procedures. The solutions may also be mixed to form combination remedies of several or all of the gems.

The following gems are used in gem therapy and will be found most useful in the treatment of the chakras.

Ruby, carrying the red cosmic ray, is used in the treatment of anaemia, circulatory problems, physical debility, common colds and states of collapse. Those individuals classified as mentally retarded respond well to the red ray.

Pearl, giving off the orange cosmic ray, is used for treating cases of gout, rheumatic conditions, asthma, gall stones, certain inflammatory states and menopause imbalances.

Coral, with its yellow cosmic rays, is used to treat stomach ailments, liver disease, diabetes, eczema and other skin troubles, haemorrhoids and nervous exhaustion.

Emerald, releases the cooling green cosmic rays which are used to treat influenza, syphilis, headaches, neuralgias, cancer, skin problems, hypertension, heart trouble and ulcers.

Moonstone, the blue cosmic ray, works well in the treatment of any conditions related to the throat chakra, such as asthma, laryngitis and coughs. It is also excellent for chickenpox, measles, scarlet fever, typhoid, and smallpox. Headaches, insomnia, shock, stings and burns all respond well to this colour.

Diamond which carries the indigo cosmic ray, is used for treating eye problems, whooping cough, certain forms of paralysis, obsession, purulent tonsils, delirium tremens and infantile convulsions.

Sapphire, concentrates within it the violet cosmic ray which

is used to treat nervous and mental disorders, epilepsy, con-
cussion, certain tumours, skin ulcers and neuralgia.

There are two other gems which are frequently used, the
first being *onyx* which carries the ultra-violet frequency; this is
used for rheumatic conditions, liver disease, smallpox and in
the treatment of any bacterial or viral infection. The other
gem is *cat's eye*; this is found at the other end of the spectrum
giving off the infrared rays. It is used for skin diseases, disorders of the uterus, headaches, indigestion and asthma.

Each gem, carrying as it does the cosmic colour frequency
assigned to it, may be used in the treatment of a variety of
conditions. Those listed are simply a guide. The rule to remember is that each patient and each disease is an individual
entity, therefore no hard and fast rules can be laid down as to
their use. This must be determined by the practitioner through
the radionic instrument.

Apart from the Bach and gem remedies, the centre therapist
also utilizes a wide variety of homoeopathic medicines which
may be broadcast to the patient or given orally. The subject of
homoeopathy is too vast to cover in this book, but in the
main, most radionic practitioners have a working knowledge of
a limited number of the medicines available, and should thus
be able to apply this knowledge in the treatment of the
chakras by way of the radionic instrument.

CHAPTER TEN

THE FUTURE TREND

After two years of using our radio instruments, we found in a deeper study of ancient wisdom amazing and satisfying corroboration of our own development of rates of vibration.

Ruth Drown, D.C.

Remarkable work has been done in the field of radionics since the de la Warr laboratories carried forward the torch lit by the physicians Abrams and Drown. Instruments have been refined and modified and new concepts built in. Energraphs taken on the de la Warr radionic camera have revealed the formative force fields that underlie the physical form, and a vast amount of clinical evidence has been amassed to bear witness to the efficacy of radionic therapy.

Despite this essential consolidation of the work of Abrams and Drown, I feel that the 'golden thread' running through it has passed unnoticed. Even the most cursory examination of these pioneers clearly shows that from physical beginnings they were heading rapidly towards the more esoteric aspects of healing at a distance by instrumental means.

The physical approach reached its high point when Ruth Drown placed the emphasis of radionic diagnosis and treatment upon the endocrine gland system. Not content with this, she showed quite conclusively that the healing art of radionics was directly related to a knowledge of man and nature as outlined in the ancient metaphysical teachings.

Each patient, she said, is a cell within the body of this vast Life in which we live and move and have our being. And it is the radionic practitioner's role to bring that 'cell' from a state of dis-ease, back to a harmonic *rapport* with the Divine Life.

If a radionic practitioner is to intercede on behalf of a patient, and utilize the healing forces present in the cosmos, it can only be done on a solid basis of knowledge relevant to·the subtle aspects of man and nature, and not on the basis of the physical organic systems which are at the heart of the present trend.

Where it may have been necessary to approach radionics in a physical manner, it is now time to move into the relatively uncharted waters of the human force fields — to study the action of the chakras and to understand their role in harmonizing and maintaining the physical body, thus simplifying and increasing the effectiveness of this healing therapy.

Radionics has a unique intrinsic quality that enables it to act as a bridge between the physical and subtle aspects of nature, and as such it has the potential to bear witness to the occult anatomy of man. It remains for practitioners to recognise this fact and to act upon the implications. To this end this brief introduction to radionics and the subtle anatomy of man has been written.

These books are useful in the further study of radionics and its relationship to the subtle anatomy of man and healing.

Matter in the Making by Langston Day & George de la Warr. Vincent Stuart Ltd.

An Introduction to Medical Radiesthesia and Radionics by Vernon Wethered. C.W. Daniel Co. Ltd.

New Light on Therapeutic Energies, by Mark Gallert, N.D. James Clarke & Co. Ltd.

Gem Therapy (Revised Edition) by Dr. B. Bhattacharya. Firma K.L. Mukhopadhyay.

Healing by I. and G. Cooke. White Eagle Publishing Trust.

Esoteric Healing by Alice A. Bailey. Lucis Press.

Treatise on Cosmic Fire by Alice A. Bailey. Lucis Press.

The Soul and its Mechanism by Alice A. Bailey. Lucis Press.

Physical and Ethereal Spaces by George Adams. Steiner Press.

Bach Flower Remedies by Nora Weeks and Victor Bullen. C.W. Daniel Co. Ltd.

The Pattern of Health by Dr. A. Westlake. Vincent Stuart Ltd.

Life Threatened and Way Out by Dr. Aubrey Westlake. Vincent Stuart Ltd.

Breakthrough To Creativity by Dr. Shafica Karagula

For further information about Radionics please contact
    The Secretary
    The Radionic Association
    Baerlein House
    Goose Green
    Deddington
    Oxford OX15 0SZ